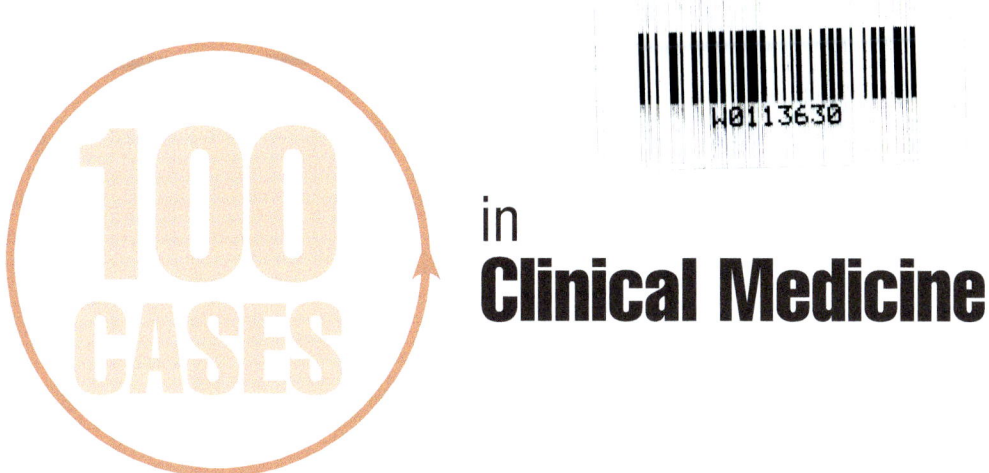

in
Clinical Medicine

100 Cases in Clinical Medicine presents 100 scenarios commonly seen by medical students and junior doctors in the emergency or outpatient department, on the ward or in the community setting. Each case begins with a succinct summary of the patient's history, examination and initial investigation. The text includes photographs where relevant and questions on the diagnosis and management of each case. The answers provide a detailed discussion on each topic, with further illustration where appropriate. Most of the cases included are common problems, but the book also includes more unusual cases to illustrate specific points and to emphasise that rare things do present occasionally and to prepare the student or trainee for these. The cases are arranged within clinical systems and specialties, though of course there may be significant overlap between these since symptoms such as breathlessness and pain may relate to many different clinical problems in various systems.

Making speedy and appropriate clinical decisions, and choosing the best course of action to take as a result, are the most important and challenging parts of training to be a doctor. These true-to-life cases will teach students and junior doctors to recognise important clinical symptoms and signs and to develop the diagnostic and management skills needed for the cases they will encounter on the job.

100 Cases
About the Series

Making speedy and appropriate clinical decisions and choosing the best course of action to take as a result is one of the most important and challenging parts of training to become a doctor. The real-life cases presented in the 100 Cases series encompass emergency, ward, and outpatient and community scenarios, and have been designed specifically to help medical students and junior doctors to develop their diagnostic and management skills.

100 Cases in Dermatology
Rachael Morris-Jones, Ann-Marie Powell, Emma Benton

100 Cases in Radiology
Robert Thomas, James Connelly, Christopher Burke

100 Cases in Orthopaedics and Rheumatology
Parminder J Singh, Catherine Swales

100 Cases in Surgery, 2E
James Gossage, Bijan Modarai, Arun Sahai, Richard Worth, Kevin G Burnand

100 Cases in Clinical Ethics and Law, 2E
Carolyn Johnston, Penelope Bradbury

100 Cases in Paediatrics, 2E
Ronny Cheung, Aubrey Cunnington, Simon Drysdale, Joseph Raine, Joanna Walker

100 Cases in General Practice, 2E
Anne E. Stephenson, Martin Mueller, John Grabinar

100 Cases in Psychiatry, 2E
Barry Wright, Subodh Dave, Nisha Dogra

100 Cases in Emergency Medicine and Critical Care
Eamon Shamil, Praful Ravi, Dipak Mistry

100 Cases in Clinical Pharmacology, Therapeutics and Prescribing
Kerry Layne, Albert Ferro

100 Cases in Acute Medicine, 2E
Henry Fok, Kerry Layne, Adam Nabeebaccus

100 Cases in Clinical Pathology and Laboratory Medicine, 2E
Eamon Shamil, Praful Ravi, Ashish Chandra

100 Diagnostic Dilemmas in Clinical Medicine, 2E
Kerry Layne

100 Cases in Obstetrics and Gynaecology, 3E
Cecilia Bottomley, Ruth MacSwan, Janice Rymer

100 Cases in Clinical Medicine, 4E
Eamon Shamil, Praful Ravi

For more information about this series please visit: https://www.routledge.com/100-Cases/book-series/CRCONEHUNCAS

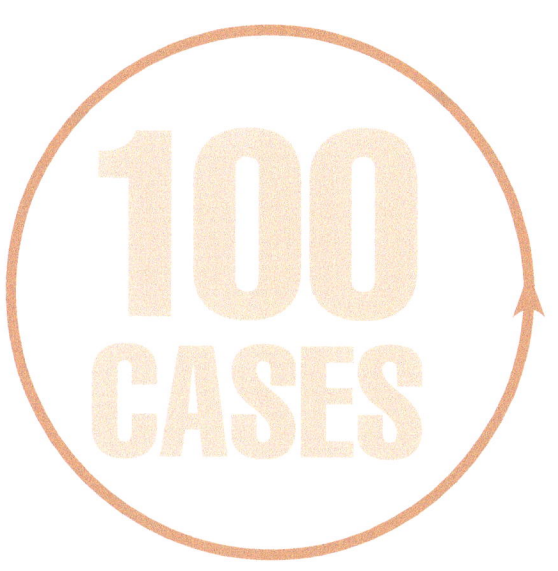

100 CASES

Fourth Edition

in

Clinical Medicine

Eamon Shamil MBBS MRes MRCS DOHNS FRCS (ORL-HNS)
Locum Consultant ENT Surgeon
Imperial College Healthcare NHS Trust
London, England

Praful Ravi MA MBBChir MRCP
Dana-Farber Cancer Institute
Assistant Professor, Harvard Medical School
Boston, USA

100 Cases Series Editor:
Janice Rymer MBBS FRACP
Professor of Obstetrics & Gynaecology and Dean
of Student Affairs, King's College London School
of Medicine, London, UK

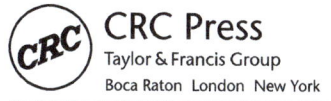

CRC Press

Taylor & Francis Group
Boca Raton London New York

CRC Press is an imprint of the
Taylor & Francis Group, an **informa** business

Designed cover image: Getty Images®. Credit: mixetto.

Fourth edition published 2026
by CRC Press
2385 NW Executive Center Drive, Suite 320, Boca Raton FL 33431

and by CRC Press
4 Park Square, Milton Park, Abingdon, Oxon, OX14 4RN

CRC Press is an imprint of Taylor & Francis Group, LLC

© 2026 Eamon Shamil and Praful Ravi

First edition published by Arnold 2000; Third edition published by CRC Press 2014

This book contains information obtained from authentic and highly regarded sources. While all reasonable efforts have been made to publish reliable data and information, neither the author[s] nor the publisher can accept any legal responsibility or liability for any errors or omissions that may be made. The publishers wish to make clear that any views or opinions expressed in this book by individual editors, authors or contributors are personal to them and do not necessarily reflect the views/opinions of the publishers. The information or guidance contained in this book is intended for use by medical, scientific or health-care professionals and is provided strictly as a supplement to the medical or other professional's own judgement, their knowledge of the patient's medical history, relevant manufacturer's instructions and the appropriate best practice guidelines. Because of the rapid advances in medical science, any information or advice on dosages, procedures or diagnoses should be independently verified. The reader is strongly urged to consult the relevant national drug formulary and the drug companies' and device or material manufacturers' printed instructions, and their websites, before administering or utilizing any of the drugs, devices or materials mentioned in this book. This book does not indicate whether a particular treatment is appropriate or suitable for a particular individual. Ultimately, it is the sole responsibility of the medical professional to make his or her own professional judgements, so as to advise and treat patients appropriately. The authors and publishers have also attempted to trace the copyright holders of all material reproduced in this publication and apologize to copyright holders if permission to publish in this form has not been obtained. If any copyright material has not been acknowledged please write and let us know so we may rectify in any future reprint.

Except as permitted under U.S. Copyright Law, no part of this book may be reprinted, reproduced, transmitted, or utilized in any form by any electronic, mechanical, or other means, now known or hereafter invented, including photocopying, microfilming, and recording, or in any information storage or retrieval system, without written permission from the publishers.

For permission to photocopy or use material electronically from this work, access www.copyright.com or contact the Copyright Clearance Center, Inc. (CCC), 222 Rosewood Drive, Danvers, MA 01923, 978-750-8400. For works that are not available on CCC please contact mpkbookspermissions@tandf.co.uk

Trademark notice: Product or corporate names may be trademarks or registered trademarks and are used only for identification and explanation without intent to infringe.

ISBN: 9781032396958 (hbk)
ISBN: 9781032363790 (pbk)
ISBN: 9781003350934 (ebk)

DOI: 10.1201/9781003350934

Typeset in Baskerville
by KnowledgeWorks Global Ltd.

To our parents and our teachers

Eamon Shamil and Praful Ravi

CONTENTS

Section 4: Cardiology

Section 5: Endocrinology

Section 6: Haematology

Section 7: Respiratory

Section 8: Nephrology

Section 9: Infectious Diseases and Microbiology

Section 10: Gastroenterology

ABBREVIATIONS

AAT	alanine aminotransferase
ACE	angiotensin-converting enzyme
AchE	acetylcholinesterase
ACS	acute coronary syndrome
ACTH	adrenocorticotrophic hormone
AD	Alzheimer's disease
AF	atrial fibrillation
AIDS	acquired immune deficiency syndrome
ALT	alanine aminotransferase
AML	acute myeloid leukaemia
ANCA	antineutrophilic cytoplasmic antibodies
ARAS	atherosclerotic renal artery stenosis
AST	aspartate aminotransferase
AV	atrioventricular
AVC	arrhythmogenic ventricular cardiomyopathy
AVP	arginine vasopressin
AVRT	atrio-ventricular re-entry tachycardia
BCG	bacille Calmette–Guérin
BMI	body mass index
CABG	coronary artery bypass graft
CAP	community acquired pneumonia
CCS	Canadian Cardiovascular Society
CK	creatine kinase
CMV	cytomegalovirus
COPD	chronic obstructive pulmonary disease
CPAP	continuous positive airway pressure
CPR	cardiopulmonary resuscitation
CPVT	catecholaminergic polymorphic ventricular tachycardia
CRP	C-reactive protein
CRT	cardiac resynchronisation therapy
CSF	cerebrospinal fluid
CT	computed tomography
CTPA	computed tomographic pulmonary angiography
CVP	central venous pressure
DC	direct current (cardioversion)
DDAVP	l-deamino-8-d-arginine vasopressin
DEXA	dual-energy X-ray absorptiometry
DILI	drug-induced liver injury
DOT	directly observed therapy
EBV	Epstein–Barr virus
ECG	electrocardiogram
EEG	electroencephalogram
EMG	electromyogram
ERCP	endoscopic retrograde cholangiopancreatography
ESR	erythrocyte sedimentation rate
FENO	fractional exhaled nitric oxide
FER	forced expiratory ratio

FEV$_1$	forced expiratory volume in 1 s
FIT	faecal immunochemical test
FMD	fibromuscular dysplasia
FVC	forced vital capacity
G6PD	glucose-6-phosphate dehydrogenase
GAS	group A *Streptococcus*
GCS	Glasgow Coma Scale
GFR	glomerular filtration rate
GP	general practitioner
GPA	granulomatosis with polyangiitis
GTN	glyceryl trinitrate
HbA$_{1c}$	haemoglobin A$_{1c}$
HbF	haemoglobin F
HBV	hepatitis B virus
HCC	hepatocellular carcinoma
HIV	human immunodeficiency virus
5-HIAA	5-hydroxyindole acetic acid
5-HT	5-hydroxytryptamine
IBS	irritable bowel syndrome
ICD	implantable cardioverter-defibrillator
ICU	intensive care unit
IgA	immunoglobulin A
IgG	immunoglobulin G
IgM	immunoglobulin M
iNOS	inducible nitric oxide synthase
INR	international normalised ratio
IPF	idiopathic pulmonary fibrosis
IVIG	intravenous immunoglobulin
JVP	jugular venous pressure
LABA	long-acting beta-agonist
LMWH	low-molecular-weight heparin
LP	lumbar puncture
LQTS	long QT syndrome
LTRA	leukotriene receptor antagonist
MACE	major adverse cardiovascular events
MAS	mandibular advancement splints
MRCP	magnetic resonance cholangiopancreatography
MRI	magnetic resonance imaging
MCV	mean corpuscular volume
MMSE	Mini-Mental State Examination
MRSA	methicillin-resistant *Staphylococcus aureus*
MSSA	methicillin-sensitive *Staphylococcus aureus*
NAD	nothing abnormal detected
NO	nitric oxide
NSAID	non-steroidal anti-inflammatory drug
NSIP	non-specific interstitial pneumonitis
NSU	non-specific urethritis
OSA	obstructive sleep apnoea
PaCO$_2$	arterial partial pressure of carbon dioxide
P$_a$o$_2$	pressure of arterial oxygen

PBC	primary biliary cholangitis
PCI	percutaneous coronary intervention
pco$_2$	partial pressure of carbon dioxide
PEF	peak expiratory flow
PET	positron-emission tomography
po$_2$	partial pressure of oxygen
PTH	parathormone
RV	right ventricle/ventricular
SABA	short-acting β2-agonist
SAH	subarachnoid haemorrhage
SAMA	short-acting muscarinic antagonist
SIADH	syndrome of inappropriate ADH secretion
SLE	systemic lupus erythematosus
STEMI	ST-elevation myocardial infarction
SVT	supraventricular tachycardia
T4	thyroxine
TB	tuberculosis
TIA	transient ischaemic attack
TIBC	total iron-binding capacity
TNF	tissue necrosis factor
TSH	thyroid-stimulating hormone
TPO	thyroid peroxidase
UIP	usual interstitial pneumonia
VDRL	venereal disease research laboratory
VF	ventricular fibrillation
VSD	ventricular septal defect
VT	ventricular tachycardia
WB-MRI	Whole-body MRI
WPW	Wolff-Parkinson-White

PREFACE

It has been our great privilege to be invited to take on the editorial role for the fourth edition of *100 Cases in Clinical Medicine*, which is undoubtedly the flagship in the 100 Cases series. As medical students, we recall using prior editions of this book, with its concise presentation of the case vignette leading on to a discussion of the differential diagnoses and broader topic at hand being ideal preparation for clinical examinations and finals.

While there is no substitute for learning medicine 'on the wards' or 'in the clinic', no student could possibly ever see all the major (and minor) medical conditions or diseases that they may be confronted with in everyday clinical practice. Moreover, in today's world, patients are rarely as 'straightforward' as may be presented in the textbooks and there is often no one unifying diagnosis. The role of this book is to highlight common clinical scenarios in clinical medicine and encourage the reader to think about the underlying pathophysiology and generate a list of potential diagnoses, and then to lead them towards why one (or two) diagnosis (diagnoses) may be most likely. This captures the essence of modern medicine.

We hope that you enjoy working through these cases and that they help formulate a way of thinking through clinical scenarios, which you may be able to take forward into your medical careers.

ACKNOWLEDGEMENTS

We thank the following for their respective contributions to the Cases in this Fourth Edition:

Dr Deena Seennapen BSc MBBS
UCL Medical School

Dr Edd Maclean MBBS BSc MRCP AKC
Specialist Registrar in Cardiology

Dr Akish Luintel MBBS BSc MRCP DTMH
Specialist Registrar in Infectious Diseases and Internal Medicine

Dr Conor Bowman MBChB MA MRCP FRCPath DTM DipHIV PGCCE AFHEA
Specialist Registrar in Infectious Diseases and Medical Microbiology

Dr Tsz Ki Ko MBChB BSc PgCert
Department of Respiratory Medicine, County Hospital, Stafford

Miss Denise Jia Yun Tan MBChB BSc MMed MRCS (ENT)
Core Surgical Trainee, West Midlands Deanery

We also thank Miss Sophia Elpida Doran for her assistance.

Section 1
HEPATOLOGY

CASE 1: NAUSEA AND WEIGHT LOSS

History

A man of 45 consults his general practitioner (GP) with a 6-month history of reduced appetite and weight loss, from 78 kg to 71 kg. During the past 3 months, he has had intermittent nausea, especially in the mornings, which has been accompanied by vomiting on several occasions. For 1 month, he has noted swelling of his ankles. Despite his weight loss, he has recently noticed his trousers getting tighter. He has had no abdominal pain. He has no relevant past history and knows no family history as he was adopted. He takes no medication. From the age of 18, he has smoked 5–6 cigarettes daily and drunk 15–20 units of alcohol per week. He has been a chef all his working life. He now lives alone as his wife left him 1 year ago.

Examination

He has plethoric features and pitting oedema of his ankles. He has nine spider naevi on his upper trunk. His pulse rate is 92/min. His jugular venous pressure (JVP) is not raised, and his blood pressure is 146/84 mmHg. The cardiovascular and respiratory systems are normal. The abdomen is distended. He has no palpable masses, but there is shifting dullness and a fluid thrill.

🔍 INVESTIGATIONS

		Normal
Haemoglobin	12.6 g/dL	13.3–17.7 g/dL
Mean corpuscular volume (MCV)	107 fL	80–99 fL
White cell count	10.2×10^9/L	$3.9–10.6 \times 10^9$/L
Platelets	121×10^9/L	$150–440 \times 10^9$/L
Sodium	131 mmol/L	135–145 mmol/L
Potassium	4.2 mmol/L	3.5–5.0 mmol/L
Urea	2.2 mmol/L	2.5–6.7 mmol/L
Creatinine	101 µmol/L	70–120 µmol/L
Calcium	2.44 mmol/L	2.12–2.65 mmol/L
Phosphate	1.2 mmol/L	0.8–1.45 mmol/L
Total protein	48 g/L	60–80 g/L
Albumin	26 g/L	35–50 g/L
Bilirubin	25 mmol/L	3–17 mmol/L
Alanine transaminase	276 IU/L	5–35 IU/L
Gamma-glutamyl transaminase	873 IU/L	11–51 IU/L
Alkaline phosphatase	351 IU/L	30–300 IU/L
International normalised ratio (INR)	1.4	0.9–1.2

Urinalysis: no protein; no blood

❓ QUESTIONS

- What are your interpretations of the findings?
- What is the diagnosis?
- How would you manage this patient?

ANSWER 1

This man has signs of chronic liver disease with ascites and oedema. The number of spider naevi is more than the accepted normal of 3. The most common cause of chronic liver disease is alcohol. He is at increased risk of alcohol misuse because he works in the catering industry. His symptoms of morning nausea and vomiting are typical of alcohol misuse. Chronic alcohol excess would account for his cushingoid appearance due to the increases of adrenocorticotrophic hormone (ACTH) secretion. Macrocytic anaemia can be due to dietary folate deficiency or the direct toxic action of alcohol on the bone marrow. The rise in bilirubin is insufficient to cause jaundice. The low serum albumin and raised INR may be due to impaired synthetic function of clotting factors produced by the liver. Thrombocytopenia may be from platelet sequestration in an enlarged spleen as a result of portal hypertension from liver cirrhosis.

However, his alcohol intake is too low to be consistent with the diagnosis of alcoholic liver disease. When the provisional diagnosis is discussed with him, though, he eventually admits that his alcohol intake has been at least 40–50 units per week for the past 20 years. His alcohol intake has increased further during the past year after his marriage had ended.

Differential diagnosis includes chronic viral hepatitis B or C, metabolic inherited conditions such as Wilson's disease, haemochromatosis and alpha-1-antitrypsin deficiency, and autoimmune hepatitis. These conditions should be considered in a patient without any history of significant alcohol intake. Further investigations include the measurement of hepatitis viral serology, ferritin, copper studies, alpha-1-antitrypsin deficiency and liver autoantibodies. These tests were negative in this case. Ultrasound of the abdomen showed moderate ascites, a slight reduction in liver size and an increase in splenic length of 2–3 cm, indicating that portal hypertension has developed.

The crucial aim in management is to counsel the patient on the necessity to stop drinking alcohol and signpost to support through an alcohol addiction unit. Acute management should include an alcohol withdrawal regimen with diazepam or chlordiazepoxide to reduce the risk of withdrawal seizures. Attention needs to be paid to nutrition. Intravenous thiamine should be given to prevent Wernicke's encephalopathy. Vitamin K is used to correct clotting abnormalities. An ascitic tap should be performed to exclude spontaneous bacterial peritonitis (which may be asymptomatic). Treatment of ascites includes a low-sodium diet and spironolactone. Daily weights should be used to measure fluid losses. Surveillance endoscopy and banding of oesophageal varices should be considered in this patient, as there is evidence of portal hypertension. If oesophageal varices are present, a non-selective beta-blocker such as carvedilol can be used to reduce portal hypertension and prevent variceal formation.

 KEY POINTS

- Patients who drink excessive amounts of alcohol will often disguise this fact in their history.
- Alcoholic liver disease has a poor prognosis if the alcohol intake is not terminated.

CASE 2: ANOREXIA AND FEVER

History

A 22-year-old man presented with malaise and anorexia for 1 week. He vomited on one occasion, with no blood. He has felt feverish but has not taken his temperature. For 2 weeks, he has had aching pains in the knees, elbows and wrists without any obvious swelling of the joints. He has not noticed any change in his urine or bowels.

Five years ago, he had glandular fever confirmed serologically. He smokes 25 cigarettes per day and drinks 20–40 units of alcohol per week. He has taken marijuana and ecstasy occasionally over the past 2 years and various tablets and mixtures at clubs without being sure of the constituents. He denies any intravenous drug use. He has had irregular homosexual contacts but says that he has always used protection. He claims to have had an HIV test that was negative 6 months earlier. He has not travelled abroad in the past 2 years.

He is unemployed and lives in a flat with three other people. There is no relevant family history.

Examination

He has a temperature of 38.6°C and looks unwell. He looks as if he may be a little jaundiced. He is a little tender in the right upper quadrant of the abdomen. There are no abnormalities to find on examination of the joints or in any other system.

🔍 INVESTIGATIONS

		Normal
Haemoglobin	14.1 g/dL	13.3–17.7 g/dL
Mean corpuscular volume (MCV)	85 fL	80–99 fL
White cell count	11.5 × 10⁹/L	3.9–10.6 × 10⁹/L
Platelets	286 × 10⁹/L	150–440 × 10⁹/L
Prothrombin time	17 s	10–14 s
Sodium	135 mmol/L	135–145 mmol/L
Potassium	3.5 mmol/L	3.5–5.0 mmol/L
Urea	3.2 mmol/L	2.5–6.7 mmol/L
Creatinine	64 µmol/L	70–120 µmol/L
Bilirubin	50 mmol/L	3–17 mmol/L
Alkaline phosphatase	376 IU/L	30–300 IU/L
Alanine aminotransferase (AAT)	570 IU/L	5–35 IU/L
Fasting glucose	4.1 mmol/L	4.0–6.0 mmol/L

❓ QUESTIONS

- What is your interpretation of the findings?
- What is the likely diagnosis?
- What treatment is required?

ANSWER 2

The diagnosis is likely to be acute viral hepatitis. The biochemical results show abnormal liver function tests with a predominant change in the transaminases, indicating a hepatocellular rather than an obstructive problem in the liver. This might be caused by hepatitis A, B, C or E. The raised white count is compatible with acute hepatitis. Homosexuality and intravenous drug abuse are risk factors for hepatitis B and C. Other viral infections, such as cytomegalovirus and herpes simplex virus, are possible. The drug ingestion history is unclear. There is a possibility of a drug-induced liver injury (DILI), and this should be considered as a differential diagnosis. However, the prodromal joint symptoms suggest a viral infection as the cause, and this is more common with hepatitis B. Serological tests can be used to see whether there are immunoglobulin M (IgM) antibodies, indicating acute infection with one of these viruses, to confirm the diagnosis. Viral loads can also be measured. The reported negative HIV test 6 months earlier makes an HIV-associated condition unlikely, although patients are not always reliable in their accounts of HIV tests. HIV seroconversion should also be considered.

This man has acute hepatitis B (HBV) infection. About 30% of cases develop jaundice. Treatment is basically supportive in the acute phase. Antiviral drugs are not indicated in the vast majority of patients with acute hepatitis B. The prothrombin time in this patient is raised slightly but not enough to be an indicator of very severe disease. The threshold for treating viral hepatitis B includes the presence of liver cirrhosis, significant derangement of the synthetic function of the liver, presence of hepatocellular carcinoma (HCC), AAT × 2 upper limit of normal and a viral DNA count >20,000, concomitant HIV and in patients on immunosuppression or due to start immunosuppression for other clinical indications. Alcohol and any other hepatotoxic drug intake should be avoided until liver function tests are back to normal. Rare complications of the acute illness are fulminant hepatic failure, aplastic anaemia, myocarditis and vasculitis. The opportunity should be taken to advise him about the potential dangers of his intake of cigarettes, drugs and alcohol and of sexually transmitted diseases and to offer him appropriate support in these areas. HBV can survive outside the body for some time and he should advise his flatmates not to share razors and toothbrushes with him. They should consider being vaccinated. Only about 5% of adults with acute hepatitis B will develop chronic infection. Hepatitis B is an oncogenic virus and can cause HCC in the absence of liver cirrhosis. Patients with alcoholic liver disease who are infected with hepatitis B have a worse liver prognosis.

 KEY POINTS

- Viral hepatitis is often associated with a prodrome of arthralgia and flu-like symptoms.
- Confirmatory evidence should be sought for patient's reports of HIV test results.
- Sexual transmission and intravenous drug use are the main methods of transmission of hepatitis B in adults in the developed world.
- Acute hepatitis B infection is a notifiable disease in the UK.

CASE 3: OVERDOSE?

History

A 30-year-old woman is brought to the emergency department at 2 pm by her husband. He is worried that she has taken some tablets in an attempt to harm herself. She has a history suggestive of depression since the birth of her son 3 months earlier. She has had some counselling since that time but has not been on any medication. On the previous evening at about 10 pm, she told her husband that she was going to take some pills and locked herself in the bathroom. Two hours later, he persuaded her to come out, and she said that she had not taken anything. They went to bed, but he has brought her now because she has complained of a little nausea, and he is worried that she might have taken something when she was in the bathroom. The only tablets in the house were aspirin, paracetamol and temazepam, which he takes occasionally for insomnia.

She complains of a little nausea, although she has not vomited. She has had a little abdominal discomfort. There is no relevant previous medical or family history of note. She worked as a social worker until 30 weeks of the pregnancy.

Examination

On examination, she is mentally alert. She says that she feels sad. Her pulse is 76/min, blood pressure is 124/78 mmHg and respiratory rate is 16/min. There is some mild abdominal tenderness in the upper abdomen, but nothing else abnormal is found.

🔍 INVESTIGATIONS

		Normal
Haemoglobin	12.7 g/dL	11.7–15.7 g/dL
Mean corpuscular volume (MCV)	87 fL	80–99 fL
White cell count	6.8×10^9/L	$3.5–11.0 \times 10^9$/L
Platelets	230×10^9/L	$150–440 \times 10^9$/L
Prothrombin time	18 s	10–14 s
Sodium	139 mmol/L	135–145 mmol/L
Potassium	3.8 mmol/L	3.5–5.0 mmol/L
Urea	4.6 mmol/L	2.5–6.7 mmol/L
Creatinine	81 µmol/L	70–120 µmol/L
Alkaline phosphatase	88 IU/L	30–300 IU/L
Alanine aminotransferase (AAT)	37 IU/L	5–35 IU/L
Gamma-glutamyl transpeptidase	32 IU/L	11–51 IU/L
Glucose	5.1 mmol/L	4.0–6.0 mmol/L

❓ QUESTIONS

- What are the key points to consider in the history?
- What drug is most likely to be the cause of the symptoms?
- What should the management be now?

ANSWER 3

It is not evident from the history if the patient herself has been asked about any tablets or other agents she has taken. This would be an important area to be sure about. Of the three agents mentioned, the only one likely to be relevant is paracetamol. Aspirin and temazepam would be likely to produce more symptoms in less than 14 h if they have been taken in significant quantity. However, the salicylate level should certainly be measured; in this case, it was not raised. In the absence of drowsiness at this time, it is not necessary to consider temazepam any further.

Paracetamol overdose causes hepatic and renal damage and can lead to death from acute liver failure. The severity of paracetamol poisoning is dose related, with a dose of 15 g being serious in most patients. Patients with pre-existing liver disease and those with a high alcohol intake may be susceptible to smaller overdoses.

The only significant abnormality on the blood tests is a slightly high prothrombin time and minimally raised AAT. The prothrombin time increase (expressed alternatively as the international normalised ratio or INR) is a signal that a paracetamol overdose is likely. It is often the first test to become abnormal when there is liver damage from paracetamol overdose. If the INR is abnormal at 24 h, then a significant problem is very likely. There are few symptoms in the first 24 h except perhaps nausea, vomiting and abdominal discomfort. This may be associated with tenderness over the liver. The liver function tests usually become abnormal after the first 24 h. Maximum liver damage, as assessed by raised liver enzymes and INR, occurs at days 3–4 after overdose. Acute liver failure may develop between days 3 and 5, and renal failure occurs in about 25% of patients with severe hepatic damage. Rarely, renal failure can occur without serious liver damage.

The paracetamol level should be measured urgently and the nomogram used to consider if treatment is required. It was found to be high in this case and above the nomogram with a level of 64 mg/L. The nomogram is not reliable if the timing of overdose is not known. It should not be used in cases of staggered paracetamol overdose. The evidence of early liver damage from the INR would suggest that treatment with acetylcysteine would be appropriate. The earlier this is used the better, but it is certainly still worthwhile 16 h after the ingestion. In this case, a level of paracetamol of 64 mg/L confirmed that treatment was appropriate and that the risk of severe liver damage was high. Further advice can always be obtained by ringing one of the national poison information services. The electrolyte, renal and liver function tests and clotting studies should be monitored carefully over the first few days and referral to a liver unit considered if there is marked liver dysfunction. Patients with fulminant hepatic failure are considered for urgent liver transplantation.

The other areas that need to be addressed in this case are the mental state and the safety and care of her son and any other children. This is a serious drug overdose. She should be seen by a psychiatrist or other appropriately trained health worker. The question of any possible risk to the baby should be evaluated before she returns home.

 KEY POINTS

- Intravenous acetylcysteine and oral methionine are effective treatments for paracetamol overdose if started early enough.
- Paracetamol levels can be used to predict problems and guide treatment if the time since overdose is known.
- Paracetamol overdose should be suspected in any patient admitted with deranged liver function tests and clotting if no obvious alternative cause is apparent.

CASE 4: ABDOMINAL PAIN

History

A 58-year-old woman consults her general practitioner (GP); she has a 2-month history of intermittent dull central epigastric pain. It has no clear relationship to eating and no radiation. Her appetite is normal, she has no nausea or vomiting and she has not lost weight. Her bowel habit is normal and unchanged. There is no relevant past or family history. She has never smoked and drinks alcohol very rarely. She has worked all her life as an infant schoolteacher. Physical examination at this time was normal, with a blood pressure of 128/72 mmHg. Investigations showed normal full blood count, urea, creatinine and electrolytes and liver function tests.

An H_2 antagonist was prescribed and follow-up advised if her symptoms did not resolve. There was slight relief at first, but after 1 month, the pain became more frequent and severe and the patient noticed that it was relieved by sitting forward. It had also begun to radiate through to the back. Despite the progressive symptoms, she and her husband went on a 2-week holiday to Scandinavia, which had been booked long before. During the second week, her husband remarked that her eyes had become slightly yellow and, a few days later, she noticed that her urine had become dark and her stools pale. On return from holiday, she was referred to a gastroenterologist.

Examination

She was found to have yellow sclerae with a slight yellow tinge to the skin. There was no lymphadenopathy and her back was normal. As before, her heart, chest and abdomen were normal.

INVESTIGATIONS		
		Normal
Haemoglobin	15.3 g/dL	11.7–15.7 g/dL
White cell count	6.2×10^9/L	$3.5–11.0 \times 10^9$/L
Platelets	280×10^9/L	$150–440 \times 10^9$/L
Sodium	140 mmol/L	135–145 mmol/L
Potassium	4.8 mmol/L	3.5–5.0 mmol/L
Urea	6.5 mmol/L	2.5–6.7 mmol/L
Creatinine	111 µmol/L	70–120 µmol/L
Calcium	2.44 mmol/L	2.12–2.65 mmol/L
Phosphate	1.19 mmol/L	0.8–1.45 mmol/L
Total bilirubin	97 mmol/L	3–17 mmol/L
Alkaline phosphatase	1007 IU/L	30–300 IU/L
Alanine aminotransferase (AAT)	38 IU/L	5–35 IU/L
Gamma-glutamyl transpeptidase	499 IU/L	11–51 IU/L

? QUESTIONS

- What is the likely diagnosis?
- What further investigations should be performed?
- How can this patient be managed?

ANSWER 4

The patient has obstructive jaundice, as indicated by the history of dark urine and pale stools and the liver function tests. The pain has two typical features of carcinoma of the pancreas: relief by sitting forward and radiation to the back. An alternative diagnosis could be gallstones, but the pain is not typical.

As with obstruction of any part of the body, the objective is to define the site of obstruction and its cause. The initial investigation was an abdominal ultrasound, which showed a dilated intrahepatic biliary tree, common bile duct and gallbladder but no gallstones. The pancreas appeared normal, but it is not always sensitive to this examination owing to its depth within the body.

Further investigation of the region at the entrance of the common bile duct into the duodenum and head of the pancreas was indicated and was undertaken by computed tomography (CT) scan. It showed a small tumour in the head of the pancreas causing obstruction to the common bile duct, but no extension outside the pancreas. No abdominal lymphadenopathy was seen. No hepatic metastases were seen on this investigation or on the ultrasound. Alternative imaging techniques include magnetic resonance cholangiopancreatography (MRCP). This is a non-contrast diagnostic examination that delineates the biliary tree. Endoscopic retrograde cholangiopancreatography (ERCP) is a therapeutic procedure to remove stones from the common bile duct or insertion of stents in cases of strictures causing obstructive jaundice.

The patient underwent partial pancreatectomy with anastomosis of the pancreatic duct to the duodenum. The jaundice was rapidly relieved. Follow-up is necessary not only to detect any recurrence but also to treat any possible development of diabetes.

 KEY POINTS

- Carcinoma of the pancreas can present with non-specific symptoms in its early stages.
- It is an important cause of obstructive jaundice.
- Patients who have had a partial removal of the pancreas are at risk of diabetes.

CASE 5: ABDOMINAL PAIN

History

A 70-year-old woman has been complaining of upper abdominal pain, which has increased over the last 3 days. It has been a general ache in the upper abdomen and there have been some more severe waves of pain. She has vomited three times in the last 24 h. On two or three occasions in the past 5 years, she has had a more severe pain in the right upper abdomen. This has sometimes been associated with feeling as if she had a fever and she was treated with antibiotics on one occasion. Her appetite is generally good, but she has been off her food over the past week. She has not lost any weight. There have been no urinary or bowel problems, but she does say that her urine may have been darker than usual for a few days and she thinks the problem may be a urinary infection.

In her previous medical history, she has had hypothyroidism and is on replacement thyroxine. She has annual blood tests to check on the dose; the last test was 3 months ago. She has had some episodes of chest pain on exercise once or twice a week for 6 months and has been given atenolol 50 mg daily and a glyceryl trinitrate spray to use sublingually as needed.

Examination

Her sclerae are yellow. Her pulse is 56/min and regular. Her blood pressure is 122/80 mmHg. There are no abnormalities in the cardiovascular system or respiratory system. She is tender in the right upper abdomen and there is marked pain when feeling for the liver during inspiration. No masses are palpable in the abdomen. She is clinically euthyroid.

🔍 INVESTIGATIONS

		Normal
Sodium	139 mmol/L	135–145 mmol/L
Potassium	4.1 mmol/L	3.5–5.0 mmol/L
Urea	6.4 mmol/L	2.5–6.7 mmol/L
Creatinine	110 µmol/L	70–120 µmol/L
Calcium	2.44 mmol/L	2.12–2.65 mmol/L
Phosphate	1.19 mmol/L	0.8–1.45 mmol/L
Total bilirubin	83 mmol/L	3–17 mmol/L
Alkaline phosphatase	840 IU/L	30–300 IU/L
Alanine aminotransferase (AAT)	57 IU/L	5–35 IU/L
Gamma-glutamyl transpeptidase	434 IU/L	11–51 IU/L
Thyroid-stimulating hormone	2.3 mU/L	0.3–6.0 mU/L

❓ QUESTIONS

- How do you interpret these findings?
- What further investigations should be considered?
- What is the appropriate management?

ANSWER 5

This woman has a 5-year history of intermittent upper abdominal pain. Her current pain has lasted longer than previous episodes and, on examination, she is jaundiced. The acute pain on inspiration while palpating in the right upper quadrant is a positive Murphy's sign of inflammation of the gallbladder. The relative bradycardia in the presence of the acute illness is likely to be related to the beta-blocker therapy (atenolol) rather than hypothyroidism or any other problem. The dark urine would fit with increased conjugated bilirubin because of biliary obstruction. The conjugated bilirubin is water soluble and excreted in the urine. Without conjugated bilirubin entering the bowel, one would expect pale stools.

Her investigations show a raised bilirubin. The AAT is slightly raised, but the main abnormalities in the liver enzymes are high values of alkaline phosphatase and gamma-glutamyl transpeptidase. This is the pattern of obstructive jaundice, which can be caused by mechanical obstruction by tumour or by gallstones or by adverse effects of some drugs (e.g., phenothiazines, flucloxacillin). The drugs she is taking are not likely causes of liver problems.

The previous episodes of pain and fever over the past 5 years are likely to have been cholecystitis secondary to gallstones. If the gallbladder were to be palpable on examination, this would suggest an alternative diagnosis of malignant obstruction, since, by this time, these previous episodes of cholecystitis would usually have caused scarring and contraction of the gallbladder. To produce obstructive jaundice, one or more of her gallstones must have moved out of the gallbladder and impacted in the common bile duct. Migration of gallstones from the gallbladder occurs in around 15% of cases.

Her thyroid condition seems to be stable and not relevant to the current problem. Her angina is indicative of coronary artery disease and needs to be considered when treatment is being planned for her gallstones. An electrocardiogram (ECG) should be part of her management.

Only a minority of gallstones are radiopaque and visible on a plain radiograph, so the next investigation should be an ultrasound of the liver and biliary tract. Ultrasound will show dilation of the biliary tree but is not so reliable for identifying common bile duct stones. Magnetic resonance cholangiopancreatography (MRCP) will delineate the biliary anatomy and clarify the site and cause of the obstruction. Endoscopic retrograde cholangiopancreatography (ERCP) is the best therapeutic tool treatment of the biliary obstruction in this case, allowing intervention by sphincterotomy and clearance of the common bile duct of stones.

🔑 KEY POINTS

- Obstructive jaundice with a dilated, palpable gallbladder is likely to be caused by carcinoma at the head of the pancreas (Courvoisier's sign).
- Obstructive jaundice causes preferential elevation of alkaline phosphatase and gamma-glutamyl transpeptidase.
- When the main rise is in alanine aminotransferase, this indicates primarily hepatocellular damage.

CASE 6: VOMITING

History

A 52-year-old man presents to the emergency department at 2 am vomiting fresh red blood. He is continuing to vomit large amounts of blood. He has no associated abdominal pain. His stools have been dark black for 48 hours.

He has a history of hypertension for which he takes atenolol. He drinks a bottle of wine a day.

Examination

He is anaemic and mildly jaundiced. There are spider naevi on his upper trunk. His pulse rate is 72/min and the blood pressure 94/55 mmHg lying down, dropping to 72/42 mmHg on standing. The spleen is palpable at 4 cm below the costal margin.

🔍 INVESTIGATIONS

		Normal
Haemoglobin	6.7 g/dL	13.3–17.7 g/dL
Mean corpuscular volume (MCV)	81 fL	80–99 fL
White cell count	8.6×10^9/L	$3.9–10.6 \times 10^9$/L
Platelets	39×10^9/L	$150–440 \times 10^9$/L
Sodium	138 mmol/L	135–145 mmol/L
Potassium	3.9 mmol/L	3.5–5.0 mmol/L
Chloride	99 mmol/L	95–105 mmol/L
Urea	5.8 mmol/L	2.5–6.7 mmol/L
Creatinine	70 µmol/L	70–120 µmol/L
Bilirubin	67 mmol/L	3–17 mmol/L
Alkaline phosphatase	344 IU/L	30–300 IU/L
Alanine aminotransferase (AAT)	64 IU/L	5–35 IU/L
Gamma-glutamyl transpeptidase	467 IU/L	11–51 IU/L

? QUESTIONS

- What is the likely diagnosis?
- What further investigation is required?
- What is the appropriate management?

DOI: 10.1201/9781003350934-7

ANSWER 6

The most likely diagnosis is a variceal bleed due to underlying chronic liver disease secondary to alcohol. He has signs of chronic liver disease and his liver function tests are consistent with this. Other causes of upper gastrointestinal bleeding in patients with liver disease include peptic ulcer disease, Mallory-Weiss tear, portal hypertensive gastropathy and gastric antral vascular ectasia. Thrombocytopenia is common in cirrhosis due to a combination of reduced thrombopoietin levels, splenic sequestration of platelets and bone marrow suppression.

The estimation of blood loss is often difficult from a patient's story. Haematemesis is a frightening symptom and the amount may be overestimated. The haemoglobin level in this case is low and there is significant postural hypotension. His pulse is not fast as he is taking a beta blocker. He has signs of chronic liver disease. This is likely to be a variceal bleed.

The patient needs to be resuscitated with transfusion via a large-bore peripheral intravenous line or a central line. Restrictive transfusion with a target Hb of 7–8 g/dL (in the absence of cardiac comorbidities) has been found to be superior to generous transfusion. Fresh frozen plasma (FFP) and platelets are needed to correct coagulopathy and thrombocytopenia, respectively. However, recent evidence suggests that FFP increases hospital stay, rebleed and mortality. Intravenous antibiotics reduce infectious complications in hospitalised cirrhotic patients. Terlipressin or octreotide reduce bleeding by reducing the splanchnic blood flow and portal pressures.

Endoscopy is required to identify the bleeding point. Bleeding oesophageal varices should be treated with oesophageal band ligation or sclerotherapy. Balloon tamponade is effective at achieving short-term haemostasis and may be used until more definitive treatment is available. Transjugular intrahepatic portosystemic shunts or surgery are reserved for patients who continue to bleed despite the above measures.

After he has been stabilised, he needs to be asked questions about his alcohol intake. He should be advised to abstain from alcohol. **CAGE** criteria consist of four questions and are commonly used as a screen for alcoholism:

- Have you felt the need to **C**ut down drinking?
- Have you ever felt **A**nnoyed by criticism of drinking?
- Have you had **G**uilty feelings about drinking?
- Did you ever take a morning **E**ye opener?

 KEY POINTS

- Acute variceal bleeds are less likely to stop spontaneously than other upper gastrointestinal haemorrhages.
- The **CAGE** questionnaire is useful as a screening tool for alcoholism.
- In some surveys, alcohol is linked directly to about 25% of acute medical admissions.

CASE 7: FATIGUE

History

A 63-year-old woman is brought into the surgery by her neighbour, who has been worried that she looks increasingly unwell. On direct questioning, she reports feeling increasingly tired for about 2 years. She has been off her food but is unclear whether she has lost any weight. She was diagnosed with hypothyroidism 8 years ago and has been on thyroxine replacement, but has not had her blood tests checked for a few years. Her other complaints are of itching for 2–3 months, but she has not noticed any rash. She says that her mouth and eyes have also felt dry.

There has been no disturbance of her bowels or urine, but she reports that her urine has been rather 'strong' lately. She is 14 years postmenopausal. There is a family history of thyroid disease and of diabetes. She does not smoke and drinks two glasses of sherry every weekend. She has taken occasional paracetamol for headaches but has been on no regular medication other than thyroxine.

Examination

Her sclerae look a little yellow and she has xanthelasma around the eyes. There are some excoriated marks from scratching on her back and upper arms. The pulse is 74/min and regular; blood pressure is 128/76 mmHg. No abnormalities are found in the cardiovascular or respiratory systems. In the abdomen, the liver is not palpable, but the spleen is felt 2 cm under the left costal margin. It is not tender.

INVESTIGATIONS

		Normal
Sodium	142 mmol/L	135–145 mmol/L
Potassium	4.2 mmol/L	3.5–5.0 mmol/L
Urea	5.6 mmol/L	2.5–6.7 mmol/L
Creatinine	84 μmol/L	70–120 μmol/L
Calcium	2.24 mmol/L	2.12–2.65 mmol/L
Phosphate	1.09 mmol/L	0.8–1.45 mmol/L
Total bilirubin	84 mmol/L	3–17 mmol/L
Alkaline phosphatase	494 IU/L	30–300 IU/L
Alanine aminotransferase	63 IU/L	5–35 IU/L
Gamma-glutamyl transpeptidase	568 IU/L	11–51 IU/L
Thyroid-stimulating hormone	1.2 mU/L	0.3–6.0 mU/L
Cholesterol	7.8 mmol/L	<5.5 mmol/L
Fasting glucose	4.7 mmol/L	4.0–6.0 mmol/L

Antinuclear antibody: +
Antimitochondrial antibody: +++
Thyroid antibodies: ++

QUESTIONS

- What is your interpretation of these findings?
- What is the likely diagnosis?
- How might this be confirmed?

DOI: 10.1201/9781003350934-8

ANSWER 7

The liver function tests show a predominantly obstructive picture with raised alkaline phosphatase and gamma-glutamyl transpeptidase, while cellular enzymes are only slightly raised. The symptoms (fatigue and pruritus) and investigations are characteristic of primary biliary cholangitis (PBC), an uncommon condition found mainly in middle-aged women. In this condition, there is chronic inflammation around the small bile ducts in the portal tracts of the liver. Fatigue is often a major factor that can impair quality of life. Itching occurs because of raised levels of bile salts and can be helped by the use of a binding agent such as cholestyramine which interferes with their reabsorption. Hypercholesterolaemia, xanthelasmata and xanthomata are common. About 25–50% of newly diagnosed patients have hyperpigmentation of the skin due to melanin deposition. The dry eyes and dry mouth may occur as part of an associated sicca syndrome. The presence of antimitochondrial antibodies in the blood is typical of PBC. These antibodies are found in 95% of cases.

Hypothyroidism might explain some of her symptoms, but the normal thyroid-stimulating hormone (TSH) level shows that her current dose of 150 μg thyroxine is providing adequate replacement. The thyroid antibodies reflect the autoimmune thyroid disease, which is associated with other autoantibody-linked conditions, such as primary biliary cirrhosis.

The diagnosis is confirmed by a liver biopsy. This should be carried out only after an ultrasound confirms that there is no obstruction of larger bile ducts. Ultrasound will help to rule out other causes of obstructive jaundice, although the clinical picture described here is typical of primary biliary cirrhosis. No treatment is known to affect the clinical course of this condition.

 KEY POINTS

- The diagnosis of primary biliary cirrhosis should be considered in a patient complaining of unexplained itching, fatigue, jaundice or unexplained weight loss.
- Symptoms such as itching have a wide differential diagnosis. Dealing with the underlying cause, wherever possible, is preferable to symptomatic treatment.

Section 2
NEUROLOGY

CASE 8: A WEAK HAND

History

A 67-year-old man is referred to a neurologist by his general practitioner (GP). His symptoms are of weakness and wasting of the muscles of his left hand. He has noticed the weakness is worse after using his hand, for example, after using a screwdriver. He has also noticed cramps in his forearm muscles. On a few occasions recently, he has felt choking sensations after taking fluids. Past medical history is notable for hypertension for 15 years and a myocardial infarction 3 years previously. His medication consists of simvastatin, aspirin and atenolol. He is a retired university lecturer. He lives with his wife and they have two grown-up children. He is a non-smoker and drinks a bottle of wine a week.

Examination

Blood pressure is 146/88 mmHg. There are no abnormalities in the cardiovascular, respiratory systems or the abdomen. There is some wasting of the muscles in the upper limbs, particularly in the left hand. There is some fasciculation in the muscles of the forearms bilaterally. Power is globally reduced in the left hand and slightly reduced in the right hand. Muscle tone is normal. The biceps and triceps jerks are brisk bilaterally. There is no sensory loss. There is slight dysarthria.

? | **QUESTIONS**

- What are some key differential diagnoses?
- What is the diagnosis?
- What is the prognosis?

ANSWER 8

This man has evidence of lower motor neurone problems in the hands with weakness, wasting and fasciculation. The most likely diagnosis is motor neurone disease. This is a degenerative disease of unknown cause that affects the motor neurones of the spinal cord, the cranial nerve nuclei and the motor cortex, and usually presents between the ages of 50 and 70 years.

Motor neurone disease is divided into five types:

1. Amyotrophic lateral sclerosis (commonest, upper and lower motor neurone)
2. Primary lateral sclerosis (upper motor neurone)
3. Progressive muscular atrophy (lower motor neurone)
4. Progressive bulbar palsy (bulbar lower motor neurone)
5. Pseudobulbar palsy (bulbar upper motor neurone)

Diagnosis can be challenging in early cases. Weakness and wasting of the muscles of one hand or arm is the most common presentation. Weakness is most marked after exertion. Painful cramps of the forearm muscles are common in the early phases of the disease. Patients may present with lower limb weakness or with dysarthria or dysphagia. The characteristic physical sign of this condition is fasciculation, which is an irregular rapid contraction of segments of muscle, caused by denervation of the muscle from a lower motor neurone lesion. As in this man, reflexes can be brisk due to loss of cortical motor neurones. There is no sensory loss.

Unfortunately, motor neurone disease is a progressive and incurable condition. Patients tend to develop a spastic weakness of the legs. Bulbar palsy causes dysarthria and dysphasia. Sphincter function is usually not affected. Intellect is generally not affected.

! DIFFERENTIAL DIAGNOSES

- **Myasthenia gravis** is associated with limb weakness worsening with fatigue.
- **Pseudobulbar palsy of cerebrovascular disease** is associated with dysphagia and dysarthria in the elderly.
- **Cervical myelopathy** is a common cause of wasting and fasciculation of the upper limbs without sensory loss.
- **Brachial plexus lesions** from trauma or invasion by an apical lung tumour (Pancoast tumour) may present with unilateral arm symptoms.
- **Motor peripheral neuropathy** causes a symmetrical pattern of weakness and reflexes are reduced.

There is no curative treatment for this condition. The mean duration of survival from presentation is between 2 and 4 years. Support must be given by a multidisciplinary team. As the disease progresses and speech deteriorates, communication may be helped by computer-linked devices. A feeding gastrostomy may be required to enable adequate calorie intake. Non-invasive ventilation can be used to help respiratory failure, but death usually occurs from bronchopneumonia.

🔑 KEY POINTS

- Motor neurone disease commonly starts with weakness and wasting of one hand.
- Fasciculation of the muscles is characteristic of this condition.
- The absence of sensory loss helps in the differential diagnosis.

CASE 9: DOUBLE VISION

History

A 43-year-old woman presents to her general practitioner (GP) complaining of double vision and difficulty holding her head up, more marked in the evenings, for the last 3 months. She has problems finishing a meal because of difficulty chewing. Her husband and friends have noticed that her voice has become quieter. She has lost about 3 kg in weight in the past 6 months. She has had no significant previous medical illnesses. She lives with her husband and three children. She is a non-smoker and drinks about 15 units of alcohol per week. She is taking no regular medication.

Examination

She looks well and examination of the cardiovascular, respiratory and abdominal systems is normal. Power in all muscle groups is grossly normal but seems to decrease after testing a movement repetitively. Tone, coordination, reflexes and sensation are normal. Bilateral ptosis is present and is exacerbated by prolonged upward gaze. Pupillary reflexes, eye movements and fundoscopy are normal.

? | **QUESTIONS**

- What is the diagnosis?
- What are the major differential diagnoses?
- How would you investigate and manage this patient?

ANSWER 9

This woman's generalised weakness is caused by myasthenia gravis. Myasthenia gravis is due to the presence of anti-acetylcholine receptor antibodies causing impaired neuromuscular transmission. It characteristically affects the external ocular, bulbar, neck and shoulder girdle muscles. Weakness is worse after repetitive movements, which cause acetylcholine depletion at the postsynaptic membrane. The onset is usually gradual. Ptosis of the upper lids is often associated with diplopia due to weakness of the external ocular muscles. Speech may become soft when the patient is tired. Symptoms are usually worse in the evenings and better in the mornings. Permanent paralysis eventually develops in some muscle groups. In severe cases respiratory weakness occurs.

> **! DIFFERENTIAL DIAGNOSES OF GENERALISED MUSCLE WEAKNESS**
>
> - **Motor neurone disease:** Suggested clinically by muscle fasciculation and later by marked muscle weakness.
> - **Muscular dystrophies:** Selective muscular weakness occurs in specific diseases (e.g., facioscapulohumeral dystrophy). There is usually a family history.
> - **Dystrophia myotonica:** This causes ptosis, wasting of the masseter, temporal and sternomastoid muscles and distal muscular atrophy. There is a characteristic facial appearance with frontal baldness, expressionless facies and sunken cheeks. There may be gonadal atrophy and mental retardation. There is usually a family history. The electromyogram (EMG) is diagnostic.
> - **Polymyositis:** This may have an acute or chronic onset. A skin rash and joint pains are common. The creatine kinase level is raised and a muscle biopsy is diagnostic.
> - **Miscellaneous myopathies:** Thyrotoxic, hypothyroid, Cushing's, alcoholic.
> - **Non-metastatic associations of malignancy:** Thymoma is associated with myasthenia gravis in 10% of cases; the Eaton-Lambert myasthenic syndrome is associated with small-cell lung carcinoma.

This patient should be investigated by a neurologist. The EMG will demonstrate fatiguability in response to repetitive supramaximal stimulation. Intravenous injection of edrophonium (Tensilon) will increase muscular power for a few minutes. Blood should be assayed for acetylcholine receptor antibodies (present in 90%). Computed tomography (CT) of the thorax should be performed to detect the presence of a thymoma or lung cancer. Corticosteroids are the drugs of first choice. Anticholinesterase drugs greatly improve muscle power but have many side effects. Thymectomy should be considered. It is most effective within 5 years of diagnosis and when there is no thymoma.

> **KEY POINTS**
>
> - Myasthenia gravis is a cause of abnormal muscular fatiguability.
> - It is caused by the presence of anti-acetylcholine receptor antibodies causing impaired neuromuscular transmission.
> - In its initial stages, it affects certain characteristic muscle groups.

CASE 10: SEIZURES

History

A 23-year-old African-Caribbean woman is admitted to the emergency department having had two tonic-clonic generalised seizures, which were witnessed by her mother. Her mother says that her daughter has been behaving increasingly strangely and has been hearing voices talking about her. Recently, she has complained of severe headaches. She has lost weight and has noticed that her hair has been falling out. She has also complained of night sweats and flitting joint pains affecting mainly the small joints of her hands and feet. She works as a bank clerk. She smokes 5–10 cigarettes per day and consumes about 10 units of alcohol per week. She takes no regular medication. She has no significant medical or psychiatric history.

Examination

She is drowsy but responsive to pain. There is no neck stiffness. Her scalp hair is thin and patchy. Her temperature is 38.5°C. She has numerous small palpable lymph nodes. Her pulse rate is 104/min and regular, blood pressure is 164/102 mmHg. Examination of her cardiovascular, respiratory and abdominal systems is otherwise normal. Neurological examination reveals no focal abnormality and no papilloedema.

🔍 INVESTIGATIONS

		Normal
Haemoglobin	7.2 g/dL	11.7–15.7 g/dL
Mean corpuscular volume (MCV)	85 fL	80–99 fL
White cell count	2.2×10^9/L	$3.5–11.0 \times 10^9$/L
Platelets	72×10^9/L	$150–440 \times 10^9$/L
Erythrocyte sedimentation rate (ESR)	90 mm/h	<10 mm/h
Sodium	136 mmol/L	135–145 mmol/L
Potassium	4.2 mmol/L	3.5–5.0 mmol/L
Urea	16.4 mmol/L	2.5–6.7 mmol/L
Creatinine	176 µmol/L	70–120 µmol/L
Glucose	4.8 mmol/L	4.0–6.0 mmol/L
Lumbar puncture		
Leucocytes	150/mL	<5/mL
Cerebrospinal fluid (CSF) protein	1.2 g/L	<0.4 g/L
CSF glucose	4.1 mmol/L	<70% plasma glucose value

Urinalysis: +++ protein; +++ blood
Urine microscopy: ++ red cell; red cell casts present
Chest radiograph: normal
Electrocardiogram (ECG): sinus tachycardia
Computed tomography (CT) of the brain: normal
CSF Gram stain: negative

❓ QUESTIONS

- What is the likely diagnosis?
- How would you investigate this patient?
- How would you manage this patient?

DOI: 10.1201/9781003350934-12

ANSWER 10

This patient has a number of important symptoms, particularly the generalised seizures, auditory hallucinations, fever, arthralgia and alopecia. Investigations show low haemoglobin, raised ESR white cells and platelets with impaired renal function and blood, protein and cells in the urine. The CSF contains white cells and a high protein content but no organisms. This is a multisystem disease, and the symptoms and investigations are explained best by a diagnosis of systemic lupus erythematosus (SLE).

SLE is an autoimmune condition that is about nine times more common in women than men and is especially common in African-Caribbean and Asian individuals. It varies in severity, from a mild illness causing a rash or joint pains, to a life-threatening multisystem illness. In the brain, SLE causes small-vessel vasculitis and can present with depression, a schizophrenia-like psychosis, seizures, chorea and focal cerebral/spinal cord infarction. Common clinical presentations include a malar flush (butterfly-shaped) rash over cheeks and nose, which usually occurs after sun exposure, recent onset of photosensitivity, discoid lupus, fatigue, weight loss, fever, arthralgia, oral ulcers, Raynaud's phenomenon, lymphadenopathy, abdominal pain, diarrhoea and vomiting. Diagnosis for SLE can be complex and the varied symptoms presenting may be similar to other connective-tissue disorders.

Investigations may show leucopenia and thrombocytopenia which are common. Coombs-positive haemolytic anaemia may occur. Lumbar puncture usually shows a raised leucocyte count and protein level. Plain radiographs of affected joints (such as hands and feet) may show inflammation or non-erosive arthritis. MRI will show vasculitic lesions in the brain. Glomerulonephritis is another common manifestation of SLE and may present with microscopic haematuria/proteinuria, nephrotic syndrome or renal failure. Arthritis commonly affects the proximal interphalangeal and metacarpophalangeal joints and wrists, usually as arthralgia without any deformity.

!   **DIFFERENTIAL DIAGNOSIS OF THE COMBINATION OF HEADACHES/PSYCHIATRIC FEATURES/SEIZURES**

- Meningitis/encephalitis
- 'Recreational' drug abuse (e.g., cocaine)
- Cerebral tumour
- Acute alcohol withdrawal: Delirium tremens
- Hypertensive encephalopathy

This patient needs urgent antihypertensive treatment to lower her blood pressure and anticonvulsant treatment. Blood should be sent for antinuclear antibody (ANA) (positive in >95%), anti-DNA antibodies (present in SLE) and complement C3 and C4 levels (depressed in SLE). A renal biopsy will provide histological evidence of the severity of the lupus nephritis. Blood and urine cultures should be performed in febrile patients to exclude infection.

As soon as active infection has been excluded, treatment should be started with intravenous steroids and immunosuppressive agents such as mycophenolate and methotrexate. Rituximab or cyclophosphamide can be used in severe organ-threatening or life-threatening SLE. Intravenous immunoglobulins are used in haematological manifestations of SLE. Non-pharmacological management includes keeping a balanced diet, smoking cessation and UV sun protective measures. Support groups, counselling and cognitive behavioural therapy (CBT) can help manage the psychosocial aspect of disease. Female patients with SLE contemplating pregnancy should be advised that the disease needs to be controlled for at least 6 months prior to pregnancy, as it can lead to premature labour, miscarriage and pre-eclampsia.

 KEY POINTS

- SLE is particularly common in young African-Caribbean women.
- SLE may present with predominantly neurological or psychiatric features.
- A low white cell count or low platelet numbers are often a suggestive feature of SLE.

History

A 45-year-old woman makes an appointment to see her general practitioner (GP) because of tiredness. She has found over the past 5 weeks that she has been waking up at night with pain in the right forearm. The pain is relieved a little by taking paracetamol or ibuprofen before going to bed but it still disturbs her sleep. She has a history of mild rheumatoid arthritis, which has involved her metacarpophalangeal joints, wrists and ankles. This has been controlled since she started taking methotrexate weekly 6 months ago. Over the last week or so, she thinks the problem in her right arm is interfering with her work on the computer keyboard.

She works as a secretary and the arthritis has interfered with her work, but she has been able to return to work full time since starting the methotrexate.

She has no other relevant medical history. Her mother is on treatment for hypothyroidism and two of her sisters have type 2 diabetes. She does not smoke and drinks about 4 units of alcohol a week.

Examination

She weighs 90 kg and her height is 1.68 m. Blood pressure is 132/82 mmHg, pulse 68/min. There is no tenderness or skin abnormality at the site of the pain. She has mild ulnar deviation but no tenderness or soft-tissue swelling at the metacarpophalangeal joints. There is a little tenderness on resisted movement in both wrists. There is full pain-free movement at her elbow and shoulder joints. On neurological examination, there is diminished pinprick and two-point discrimination in the index and ring fingers of the right hand. Strength in the hand muscles is slightly limited by discomfort in the wrist but abduction of the right thumb seems weaker than other movements.

🔍 INVESTIGATIONS

		Normal
Haemoglobin	12.5 g/dL	11.7–15.7 g/dL
Mean corpuscular volume (MCV)	102 fL	80–99 fL
White cell count	8.2×10^9/L	$3.5–11.0 \times 10^9$/L
Platelets	350×10^9/L	$150–440 \times 10^9$/L
Sodium	139 mmol/L	135–145 mmol/L
Potassium	4.5 mmol/L	3.5–5.0 mmol/L
Urea	4.4 mmol/L	2.5–6.7 mmol/L
Creatinine	81 µmol/L	70–120 µmol/L
Glucose	4.8 mmol/L	4.0–6.0 mmol/L

❓ QUESTIONS

- What is the diagnosis?
- What investigations should be considered?
- What treatment would be appropriate?

DOI: 10.1201/9781003350934-13

ANSWER 11

The story of pain in the forearm at night is characteristic of carpal tunnel syndrome caused by compression of the median nerve in the carpal tunnel at the wrist. There are a number of factors in the history that could be related to the reason this woman has developed carpal tunnel syndrome. Rheumatoid arthritis is associated with carpal tunnel syndrome. It is also more likely in those who use their hands at work or other activities. Her return to work as a secretary could be relevant. Other activities such as painting or other do-it-yourself projects may provoke problems. There is a family history of hypothyroidism, which is another association. She is obese (BMI 31.9 kg/m^2), which is another risk factor for carpal tunnel syndrome. The random blood sugar suggests that she does not have type 2 diabetes as her sisters do, but it would still be sensible to suggest that she tries to lose weight. Women suffer carpal tunnel syndrome more than men. The problem may develop during pregnancy, possibly related to fluid retention.

Examination confirms some sensory problems in the distribution of the median nerve and weakness of abductor pollicis brevis in the thenar eminence, supplied by the median nerve. A careful examination is needed to differentiate carpal tunnel syndrome from other neurological problems such as T1 lesions and from weakness associated with active arthritis.

> ! **OTHER TESTS WHICH MAY HELP CONFIRM CARPAL TUNNEL SYNDROME**
>
> - **Tinel's test:** Slight percussion over the median nerve provokes tingling in the median nerve distribution.
> - **Phalen's manoeuvre:** Forced flexion at the wrist for 30–60 seconds exacerbates symptoms by increasing compression in the carpal tunnel.

The only significant abnormality in the investigations listed is the raised MCV. This might be related to hypothyroidism, so her thyroid stimulating hormone (TSH) levels should be measured. She is on methotrexate and a raised MCV is common on long-term methotrexate therapy. It may indicate folic acid deficiency and there is no indication that she takes folic acid. In addition to TSH, her folic acid, vitamin B12 and liver function should be assessed for investigation of macrocytosis.

The initial management of her carpal tunnel syndrome is to stop provocative movement temporarily and to give her splints to wear at night. This is usually effective in early cases. If the problems persist, then nerve conduction studies will confirm the site and extent of the lesion and local steroid injection or surgical decompression can be considered. In milder cases, the outlook is generally good although there may be mild residual tingling.

> 🔑 **KEY POINTS**
>
> - Carpal tunnel syndrome often presents with pain at night in the forearm.
> - Predisposing causes are hypothyroidism, rheumatoid arthritis, diabetes, acromegaly, obesity and fluid retention as well as repetitive wrist flexion activities and trauma.
> - Most cases settle without surgical intervention.

CASE 12: NAUSEA AND VERTIGO

History

A 17-year-old woman is admitted to the emergency department complaining of severe vertigo. This has developed over the past few hours, and previously she was well. She has the sensation of her surroundings spinning around her. She feels nauseated and sleepy. She does not have a headache. She has not had any previous medical illnesses. She is a non-smoker and says that she does not drink alcohol or take recreational drugs and is taking no regular medication. She lives with her parents and is due to sit her A-levels in 3 weeks. Her father suffers from epilepsy, and her mother has hypothyroidism.

Examination

She is drowsy and her speech is slurred. Her pulse rate is 64/min, blood pressure is 90/70 mmHg and respiratory rate is 12/min. Examination of her cardiovascular, respiratory and abdominal systems is otherwise normal. Her peripheral nervous system examination is normal apart from impaired coordination in both arms and legs and a staggering gait. Fundoscopy is normal. Her pupils are equal and reacting. There is a normal range of eye movements, but she has multidirectional nystagmus. Her hearing is normal, as is the rest of her cranial nerve examination.

> **? QUESTIONS**
>
> - What is the diagnosis?
> - What are the major differential diagnoses of vertigo?
> - How would you manage this patient?

ANSWER 12

The acute onset of these symptoms and signs with drowsiness in a 17-year-old girl raises the possibility of a drug overdose. Her father is epileptic and is likely to be taking anticonvulsants. The most likely explanation is that this patient has taken a phenytoin overdose, tablets that her father uses to control his epilepsy. She may have taken an overdose because of concern about her imminent exams. Excessive ingestion of barbiturates, alcohol and phenytoin all cause acute neurotoxicity manifested by vertigo, dysarthria, ataxia and nystagmus. In severe cases coma, respiratory depression and hypotension occur.

Vertigo is an awareness of disordered orientation of the body in space and takes the form of a sensation of rotation of the body or its surroundings.

 CAUSES OF VERTIGO

Peripheral lesions
Benign positional vertigo
Vestibular neuronitis
Ménière's disease
Middle-ear diseases
Aminoglycoside toxicity

Central lesions
Brainstem ischaemia
Posterior fossa tumours
Multiple sclerosis
Alcohol/drugs
Migraine, epilepsy

The duration of attacks is helpful in distinguishing some of these causes of vertigo. Benign positional vertigo lasts less than 1 minute. Attacks of Ménière's disease are recurrent and last up to 24 hours. Vestibular neuronitis does not recur but lasts several days, whereas vertigo due to ototoxic drugs is usually permanent. Brainstem ischaemic attacks occur in patients with evidence of diffuse vascular disease, and long tract signs may be present. Multiple sclerosis may initially present with an acute attack of vertigo that lasts for 2–3 weeks. Posterior fossa tumours usually have symptoms and signs of space-occupying lesions. Acoustic neuromas often present with vertigo and deafness. Migrainous attacks are often accompanied by nausea and vomiting. Temporal lobe epilepsy may also produce rotational vertigo, often associated with auditory and visual hallucinations. Central lesions produce nystagmus, which is multidirectional and may be vertical. Peripheral lesions induce a unilateral horizontal nystagmus.

The diagnosis in this case can be made by measuring plasma phenytoin levels and by asking the patient's father to check if his tablets are missing. Gastric lavage should be carried out if it is within 12 hours of ingestion of the tablets. Oral activated charcoal may be useful. The National Poisons Information Services is available to advise on treatment via the Internet database TOXBASE. Before discharge, she should be assessed and have counselling and treatment by psychiatrists specialising in adolescents.

 KEY POINTS

- Vertigo can be caused by a variety of neurological disorders.
- A careful history and examination may reveal the cause of vertigo.
- An overdose should be considered in any patient presenting with decreased consciousness level and respiratory depression.

History

A 44-year-old woman presents to her general practitioner (GP) complaining of headaches. These headaches have been present in previous years, but have now become more intense. She describes the headaches as severe and present on both sides of her head. They tend to worsen during the course of the day. There is no associated visual disturbance or vomiting. She also complains of loss of appetite and difficulty sleeping, with early morning waking. She has had eczema and irritable bowel syndrome diagnosed in the past, but these are not giving her problems at the moment. She is divorced with two children, aged 10 and 12 years, whom she looks after. She has a part-time job as an office cleaner. Her mother has recently died of a brain tumour. She smokes about 20 cigarettes per day and drinks 15 units of alcohol per week. She takes regular paracetamol or ibuprofen for her headaches.

Examination

She looks withdrawn. Her pulse is 74/min and regular; blood pressure is 118/76 mmHg. Examination of the cardiovascular, respiratory and gastrointestinal systems, breasts and reticuloendothelial system is normal. There are no abnormal neurological signs and fundoscopy is normal.

?	QUESTIONS

- What is the diagnosis?
- What are the major differential diagnoses?
- How would you manage this patient?

ANSWER 13

This patient has a chronic tension headache. This is the commonest form of headache. It occurs mainly in patients under the age of 50 years. The headache is usually bilateral, often with diffuse radiation over the vertex of the skull, although it may be more localised. The pain is often characterised as a sense of pressure on the head. Visual symptoms and vomiting do not occur. The pain is often at its worst in the evening. Patients may show symptoms of depression (this woman has biological symptoms of loss of appetite and disturbed sleep pattern). Sufferers may reveal sources of stress such as bereavement or difficulty with work. There may be an element of suggestion as in this case, with concern that she may have inherited a brain tumour from her mother. She is looking after two children alone and working part-time. A normal neurological examination is important for reassurance.

!   MAJOR DIFFERENTIAL DIAGNOSES OF CHRONIC HEADACHES

- **Classic migraine:** May be characterised by visual symptoms or aura followed within 30 mins by the onset of severe hemicranial throbbing, headache. Migraine without aura, often premenstrual with nausea and vomiting +/− photophobia lasting for several hours. The onset is usually in early adult life, and a positive family history may be present.
- **Cluster headaches:** The pain is unilateral, usually orbital and severe in nature. Associated with watery and bloodshot eyes, lid swelling, lacrimation, facial flushing, rhinorrhoea, mitosis +/− ptosis. It characteristically occurs 1–2 h after sleeping, lasts 1–2 h and recurs nightly for 4–12 weeks. Mainly affects men.
- **Headache caused by a space-occupying lesion (such as tumour or abscess):** Often, the headache is initially mild, but over a few weeks becomes severe and is exacerbated by coughing or sneezing. The headache is usually worse on waking, lying down and leaning forward and is associated with vomiting. There will often be other signs, including seizures, personality change and focal neurological signs.
- **Miscellaneous causes:** Sinusitis, dental disorders, cervical spondylosis, glaucoma, post-traumatic headache.

It is important to come to a clear diagnosis and to address the patient's beliefs and concerns about the symptoms. In some circumstances, it may be necessary to perform a computed tomography (CT) head scan for reassurance. Consider exploring anxiety disorders and depression in patients with chronic tension headaches.

 KEY POINTS

- Tension headaches occur mainly in those aged under 50, and patients often show features of depression.
- Tension headache should be diagnosed after other causes have been excluded.

CASE 14: HEADACHE AND CONFUSION

History

A 55-year-old man is admitted to hospital with a headache and confusion. He has a cough and a temperature of 38.2°C. He does not complain of any other symptoms. Two months earlier, he was admitted with a productive cough, and acid-fast bacilli were found in the sputum on direct smear. He had lost weight and complained of occasional night sweats. He found a place in a local hostel for the homeless and after being discharged after 1 week in hospital on antituberculous treatment with rifampicin, isoniazid, ethambutol and pyrazinamide together with pyridoxine. His chest radiograph at the time was reported as showing probable infiltration in the right upper lobe. He had a head injury 10 years previously. He smokes 15 cigarettes a day and drinks 40–60 units of alcohol each week.

Examination

He looks thin and unwell and he is slightly drowsy. His mini-mental test score is 8/10. There are some crackles in the upper zones of the chest posteriorly. His respiratory rate is 22/min. There are no neurological signs.

 INVESTIGATIONS

His chest radiograph is shown in Figure 14.1.

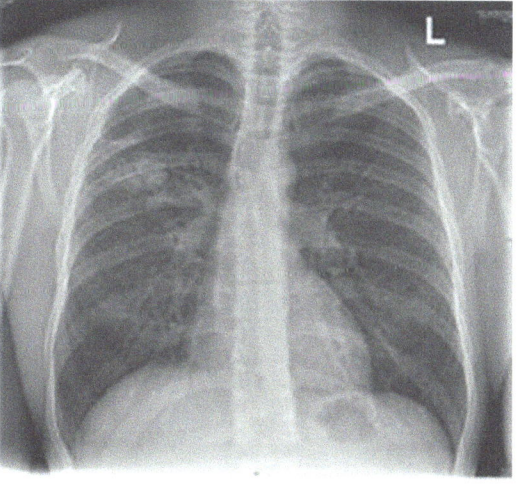

Figure 14.1 Chest radiograph.

? **QUESTIONS**

- What does the radiograph show?
- What might be the cause of his second admission?
- How should he be managed?

DOI: 10.1201/9781003350934-16

ANSWER 14

The chest radiograph shows extensive changes in the right upper zone that seem as if they are likely to be more extensive than those described at the first admission 2 months earlier. It is likely that this is a worsening of his pulmonary tuberculosis. This might have occurred because he has a resistant organism or, more likely, because he has not taken his treatment as prescribed. Risk factors for development of tuberculosis are poor nutrition, high alcohol intake and immunosuppression. Higher rates occur in those from the Indian subcontinent and parts of Africa.

The headache and confusion raise the possibility of tuberculous meningitis. Other possibilities would be liver damage from the antituberculous drugs and the alcohol, although clinical jaundice would be expected, or hyponatraemia or hypercalcaemia. If these are not present, a lumbar puncture would be indicated if there is no sign to suggest raised intracranial pressure. It would be advisable to do a computed tomography (CT) scan of the brain first since a fall related to his high alcohol consumption might have led to a subdural haemorrhage to give him his headache and confusion.

Two months since the initial finding of acid-fast bacilli in the sputum, the cultures and sensitivities of the organism should be available and checked to be sure that the organism was *Mycobacterium tuberculosis*, and that it was sensitive to the four antituberculous drugs he was given. To check compliance, blood levels of antituberculous drugs can be measured.

Comparison with his old chest radiographs showed extension of the right upper-lobe shadowing. It is difficult to be sure about activity from a chest radiograph, but extension of shadowing is obviously suspicious. 'Softer', fluffier shadowing is more likely to be associated with active disease. A direct smear of the sputum showed that acid-fast bacilli were still present on direct smear. He confirmed that he was not taking his medication regularly. His headache and confusion resolved as he stopped his high alcohol intake. Subsequently, the antituberculous therapy should be given as directly observed therapy (DOT) in a thrice-weekly regime supervised at each administration by a district nurse or health visitor.

The standard drug regimen for treating active tuberculosis without central nervous system involvement is 2 months of rifampicin, isoniazid (with pyridoxine), pyrazinamide and ethambutol, followed by 4 months of rifampicin and isoniazid (with pyridoxine). If there is central nervous system involvement, e.g., the lumbar puncture confirmed the diagnosis of tuberculous meningitis, at least 12 months of antituberculous therapy with the addition of steroids is recommended.

Common side effects of antituberculous therapy include:

- **Rifampicin:** Hepatitis, orange tears and urine, flu-like symptoms, potent liver enzyme inducer.
- **Isoniazid:** Peripheral neuropathy (prevent with pyridoxine), hepatitis, agranulocytosis, potent liver enzyme inhibitor.
- **Pyrazinamide:** Arthralgia, myalgia, hyperuricaemia causing gout, hepatitis.
- **Ethambutol:** Optic neuritis.

🔑 **KEY POINTS**

- Poor adherence to treatment regimen is the commonest cause of failure of antituberculous and other treatment.
- DOT should be used when there is any doubt about likely adherence to treatment.
- Initial polymerase chain reaction testing on sputum can predict the likelihood of resistant organisms.

CASE 15: HEADACHE

History

A 74-year-old woman presents as an emergency having suddenly developed a severe headache whilst shovelling snow in her drive. She does not recollect being taken to the hospital. The ambulance was called by the neighbours who witnessed the woman having generalised seizures. She now describes the pain as the worst headache that she has ever experienced. It is a generalised headache. She cannot tolerate bright light. She had a similar milder headache about 10 days earlier. She has a history of well-controlled hypertension. She smokes 20 cigarettes/day.

Examination

On examination she is drowsy. There is marked neck stiffness and photophobia. Blood pressure is 172/102. There are no focal neurological signs.

? | QUESTIONS

- What is the likely diagnosis?
- What are the major differential diagnoses?
- How would you investigate this patient?

ANSWER 15

A headache is one of the commonest clinical complaints. The sudden onset of a headache within seconds or a few minutes is characteristic of a subarachnoid haemorrhage (SAH). In contrast, a migraine usually takes 1 to 2 hours to reach maximal intensity. The absence of a similar headache in the past also suggests a new pathology.

Tension type headaches are the commonest headaches in the general population. The typical presentation is of mild to moderate headache, non-throbbing, bilateral with no associated symptoms. Cluster headaches are characterised by attacks of severe unilateral orbital or temporal pain, accompanied by autonomic features such as nasal congestion, lacrimation and rhinorrhoea. Migraines are often preceded by characteristic symptoms such as flashing lights and are often unilateral. Nausea and photophobia may occur during an attack. Brain tumours cause headaches by causing raised intracranial pressure. The headache is worse after coughing and is often associated with nausea and vomiting.

Patients with SAH often describe the pain as 'the worst headache in my life'. Fever associated with headache suggests an infective cause such as meningitis. A change in conscious level or personality suggests an underlying pathology. Causes: berry aneurysm rupture (80%); common sites include junctions of the posterior communicating with the internal carotid, the anterior communicating with the anterior cerebral artery or the bifurcation of the middle cerebral artery. Arterio-venous malformations (15%); rupture of an aneurysm leads to release of blood into the cerebrospinal fluid (CSF) under arterial pressure. The bleeding probably only lasts for a few seconds, but rebleeding is common. The onset of headache may be localised to the side of the aneurysm and may be associated with a brief loss of consciousness, seizure, nausea and vomiting and neck stiffness. A significant minority of patients will have a minor haemorrhage causing a sudden and severe headache (the sentinel headache) within the 3 weeks leading up to the main SAH. Physical exertion may be a trigger. Risk factors include smoking, heavy alcohol consumption, uncontrolled hypertension and a family history. Polycystic kidneys, aortic coarctation and Ehlers-Danlos syndrome are associated with berry aneurysms.

On examination, consciousness level may be reduced. There is neck stiffness and there may be pre-retinal haemorrhages. The key investigation is a non-contrast computed tomography (CT) scan. The sensitivity of a head CT for detecting blood in the CSF is highest in the first 6–12 hours, and then declines rapidly over the next few days. Lumbar puncture is essential if there is a high clinical suspicion of a SAH haemorrhage with a normal CT. The usual findings are an elevated opening pressure and an elevated red blood cell count that does not decrease after the initial few drops. Xanthochromia (red/yellow) suggests haemoglobin degradation products and is also suggestive of a recent subarachnoid haemorrhage. Once subarachnoid haemorrhage is confirmed, digital subtraction angiography is performed to identify a potential bleeding point for intervention. About 15% of patients will not have an aneurysm on angiography.

The main differential diagnoses of a SAH are a sentinel headache, cerebral venous thrombosis, acute hypertensive crisis and bacterial or viral meningitis.

SAH is associated with a mortality rate of up to 50%. Complications include rebleeding, cerebral infarction, hydrocephalus, cardiac ischaemia and hypothalamic dysfunction.

 KEY POINTS

- Sudden onset of severe headache should trigger investigation to rule out SAH.
- A sentinel headache often precedes a SAH.

CASE 16: LOSS OF CONSCIOUSNESS

History

A 52-year-old man is brought to the emergency department by ambulance. His wife recounts that while standing at a bus stop, he fell to the ground and she was unable to rouse him. His breathing seemed to stop for about 20 seconds. He then developed jerking movements affecting his arms and legs and lasting for about 2 minutes. She noticed that his face became blue and that he was incontinent of urine. He started to recover consciousness after a few minutes, although he remained drowsy with a headache. The man has not complained of any symptoms prior to this episode. There is no significant past medical history. He is a taxi driver. He smokes 20 cigarettes per day and consumes about 3 pints of beer each night.

Examination

The man looks fit and well nourished. He is afebrile. There is some bleeding from his tongue. His pulse is 84/min and regular. His blood pressure is 136/84 mmHg. Examination of his heart, chest and abdomen is normal. There is no neck stiffness, and there are no focal neurological signs. Fundoscopy is normal. His Mini-Mental State Examination (MMSE) test score is normal.

INVESTIGATIONS		
		Normal
Haemoglobin	15.6 g/dL	13.3–17.7 g/dL
Mean corpuscular volume (MCV)	85 fL	80–99 fL
White cell count	5.2×10^9/L	$3.9–10.6 \times 10^9$/L
Platelets	243×10^9/L	$150–440 \times 10^9$/L
Sodium	138 mmol/L	135–145 mmol/L
Potassium	4.8 mmol/L	3.5–5.0 mmol/L
Urea	6.2 mmol/L	2.5–6.7 mmol/L
Creatinine	76 µmol/L	70–120 µmol/L
Glucose	4.5 mmol/L	4.0–6.0 mmol/L
Calcium	2.25 mmol/L	2.12–2.65 mmol/L
Phosphate	1.2 mmol/L	0.8–1.45 mmol/L

?	QUESTIONS

- What are the differential diagnoses of this episode?
- How would you investigate and manage this patient?
- What implications does the diagnosis have for this man's livelihood?

ANSWER 16

This man has had an episode characterised as sudden onset loss of consciousness associated with the development of generalised convulsions. The principal differential diagnoses are an epileptic seizure and a syncopal (fainting) attack. Syncope is a sudden loss of consciousness due to temporary failure of the cerebral circulation. Syncope is distinguished from a seizure principally by the circumstances in which the event occurs. For example, syncope usually occurs while standing, under situations of severe stress or in association with an arrhythmia. Sometimes a convulsion and urinary incontinence occur. Thus, neither of these are specific for an epileptic attack. The key is to establish the presence or absence of prodromal symptoms. Syncopal episodes are usually preceded by symptoms of dizziness and light-headedness. Other important neurological syndromes to exclude are transient ischaemic attacks, migraine, narcolepsy and hysterical convulsions. Transient ischaemic attacks are characterised by focal neurological signs and no loss of consciousness unless the vertebrobasilar territory is affected. The onset of migraine is gradual, and consciousness is rarely lost. In narcolepsy, episodes of uncontrollable sleep may occur, but convulsive movements are absent, and the patient can be awakened.

In this man's case, the episode was witnessed by his wife, who gave a clear history of a tonic-clonic seizure. There may be warning symptoms, such as fear, or an abnormal feeling referred to some part of the body—often the epigastrium—before consciousness is lost. The muscles become tonically contracted, and the person will fall to the ground. The tongue may be bitten, and there is usually urinary incontinence. Due to spasm of the respiratory muscles, breathing ceases, and the subject becomes cyanosed. After this tonic phase, which can last up to 1 minute, the seizure passes into the clonic or convulsive phase. After the contractions end, the patient is stuporous, which lightens through a stage of confusion to normal consciousness. There is usually a post-seizure headache and generalised muscular aches.

In adults, idiopathic epilepsy rarely begins after the age of 25 years. Blood tests should be performed to exclude metabolic causes, such as uraemia, hyponatraemia, hypoglycaemia and hypocalcaemia. Blood alcohol levels and gamma-glutamyl transferase levels should also be measured as markers of alcohol abuse. A drug screen may be considered. Equally, a lumbar puncture may be indicated if infection is suspected. A computed tomography (CT) scan of the brain is needed to exclude a structural cause such as a brain tumour or cerebrovascular event. The patient should be referred to a neurologist for further investigation, including an electroencephalogram (EEG). An epilepsy diagnosis may affect the patient's ability to continue in his occupation as a taxi driver under DVLA regulations. Anti-epileptic drugs should only be commenced by a specialist, after a confirmed epilepsy diagnosis, ≥2 seizures and a detailed discussion of treatment options with the patient.

 KEY POINTS

- It is vital to get an eyewitness account of a transient neurological episode to make a diagnosis.
- New-onset epilepsy is rare in adults and should therefore be fully investigated to exclude an underlying cause.

CASE 17: MEMORY LOSS

History

An 85-year-old woman attends her general practitioner (GP) with her daughter. Her daughter says she is becoming more forgetful. On two occasions, she has left the gas on the hob. She leaves the house but then can't remember why she left. She has become lost and been returned home by the police. She used to be diligent with her finances, but recently, her daughter found piles of unpaid bills. Her mother admits she gets a bit muddled trying to add up the amounts. Her writing has deteriorated and she struggles to think of the correct words. Her daughter says her mother can remember events from her earlier life fairly well, but her short-term memory has gotten worse in the last 12 months. There has been no change in mood or appetite. There have been no hallucinations or delusions. Her mother has had no significant past medical history and has rarely needed to see doctors.

Examination

The examination of nervous, cardiovascular, respiratory and abdominal systems is entirely normal. Fundoscopy is normal. Abbreviated mental test scoring is grossly subnormal (3 out of 10).

! | **MINI-MENTAL STATE EXAMINATION (MMSE) QUESTIONNAIRE**

- What is the name of this place?
- Can you remember this address I will give to you, '42 West Street'?
- What is the time?
- What year is it?
- What is my occupation?
- How old are you?
- When is your birthday?
- What year did World War II start and end?
- Who is the name of the current monarch?
- Who was the previous prime minister?

? | **QUESTIONS**

- What is the diagnosis?
- What are the major differential diagnoses of this condition?
- How would you investigate and manage this patient?

DOI: 10.1201/9781003350934-19

ANSWER 17

The abbreviated mental test score is a screening test for cognitive impairment. The score of 3 out of 10 indicates severe impairment of cognitive function. A 30-point mini-mental state examination (MMSE) was performed and confirmed severe cognitive impairment. In this patient, the diagnosis is dementia, with gradual decline in a number of higher centre cognitive domains (language, orientation, calculation, memory).

Dementia needs to be distinguished from delirium and depression. Dementia is a progressive decline in mental ability affecting intellect, behaviour and personality. In delirium, patients are acutely confused, inattentive and often have visual hallucinations. Delirium is usually reversible once the underlying cause is addressed (commonly infection, dehydration, medication and constipation). Patients with dementia are particularly vulnerable to delirium. Depression may mimic dementia (pseudodementia), as it can cause severe retardation of cognitive, vocabulary and motor functions. Depressed patients may score poorly on the abbreviated mental state test if they are rushed. Pseudodementia from depression is reversible with antidepressant therapy.

Dementia is a syndrome that can be caused by many diseases. The commonest cause of dementia is Alzheimer's disease (AD). Progressive neuronal damage in AD occurs due to the accumulation of beta amyloid peptide with the formation of amyloid plaques and neurofibrillary tangles. Although a definitive cause is not known, studies show that causes probably include a combination of age-related changes in the brain, along with genetic, environmental and lifestyle factors. AD often begins as subtle forgetfulness and progresses over time such that patients lose their short-term memory, vocabulary and orientation. Later, long-term memory may be lost, with an inability to remember relatives' names or perform everyday tasks. In the latter stages of AD, patients may not attend to personal hygiene, diet or liquid intake. The average time of death from diagnosis is 8 to 10 years.

! CAUSES OF DEMENTIA

- Alzheimer's disease
- Multi-infarct dementia
- Frontotemporal dementia
- Vascular dementia
- Dementia with Lewy bodies
- As part of progressive neurological diseases (e.g., multiple sclerosis, Parkinson's)
- Normal-pressure hydrocephalus: dementia, ataxia, urinary incontinence
- Neurosyphilis: general paralysis of the insane
- Vitamin B12 deficiency
- Intracranial tumours; subdural haematomas
- Hypothyroidism
- AIDS dementia

The investigations in this patient should initially look for reversible causes, including a full blood count, erythrocyte sedimentation rate, serum urea and electrolytes, serum calcium, thyroid function tests, liver function tests, venereal disease research laboratory (VDRL) test for syphilis, vitamin B_{12} and folic acid, HIV serology and computed tomography (CT) of the head. In AD, the CT scan is usually normal or shows cerebral atrophy. Functional imaging such as FDG PET and SPECT may delineate subtypes where diagnosis is not clear. Detailed neurocognitive testing may be helpful to identify the cause of dementia and can be used to detect early disease.

Oral acetylcholinesterase (AchE) inhibitors such as donepezil, rivastigmine and galantamine are modestly effective in treating AD, and may delay the need for nursing home care. Memantine is an N-methyl-D-aspartate antagonist, which alone or in combination with a cholinesterase inhibitor is effective in moderate to severe AD. Special help is available in the UK for those caring for relatives with dementia. Help includes community occupational therapy, physiotherapy, a community psychiatric team, an attendance allowance, respite care, daycare or lunch clubs, priority parking and carer support groups. Specialist memory clinics offer multidisciplinary advice on treatment and support available.

 KEY POINTS

- It is important to distinguish dementia from delirium and depression.
- AD is the commonest cause of dementia.
- It may be possible to reverse or slow the progression of some types of dementia with specific treatments.

CASE 18: LEG WEAKNESS

History

A 24-year-old woman was attending her regular Sunday church service. During singing of a hymn, she suddenly fell to the ground without any loss of consciousness and told the other members of the congregation who rushed to her aid that she had complete paralysis of her left leg. She was unable to stand and was taken by ambulance to the emergency department. She has no other neurological symptoms and is otherwise healthy. She has no relevant past or family history, is on no medication and has never smoked or drunk alcohol. She works as a sales assistant in a bookshop and until recently lived in a flat with a partner of 3 years standing until they split up 4 weeks previously. She has moved back in with her parents.

Examination

She looks well and is in no distress, making light of her condition with the staff. The only abnormalities are in the nervous system. She is completely oriented and the Mini-Mental State Examination score is normal. The cranial nerves and the neurology of the upper limbs and right leg are normal. The left leg is completely still during the examination, and the patient is unable to move it on request. Tone is normal; coordination could not be tested because of the paralysis. Superficial sensation is completely absent below the margin of the left buttock and the left groin, with a clear transition to normal above this circumference at the top of the left leg. Vibration and joint position sense are completely absent in the left leg. There is normal withdrawal of the leg to nociceptive stimuli such as firm stroking of the sole and increasing compression of the Achilles' tendon. The superficial reflexes and tendon reflexes are normal, and the plantar response is flexor.

? | **QUESTIONS**

- What are the key aspects of the history?
- What is the diagnosis?
- How would you manage this case?

DOI: 10.1201/9781003350934-20

ANSWER 18

This patient has hysteria, now renamed dissociative disorder. The clues to this are the cluster of the following factors:

- The bizarre complex of neurological symptoms and signs that do not fit neuroanatomical principles (e.g., the reflex responses and withdrawal to stimuli despite the paralysis).
- The patient's lack of concern, known by the French term of *la belle indifférence*.
- The onset in relation to stress (i.e., the loss of her partner).
- Secondary gain: removing herself from the parental home, which is a painful reminder of her splitting from her partner.

None of these on its own is specific for the diagnosis, but put together, they are typical. In any case of dissociative disorder, the diagnosis is one of exclusion; in this case, the neurological examination excludes organic lesions. It is important to realise that this disorder is distinct from malingering and factitious disease. The condition is real to patients, and they must not be told that they are faking illness or wasting the time of staff.

The management is to explain the dissociation–in this case it is between her will to move her leg and its failure to respond–as being due to stress, and that there is no underlying serious disease such as multiple sclerosis. A positive attitude that she will recover is essential, and it is important to reinforce this with appropriate physical treatment, in this case physiotherapy.

The prognosis in cases of recent onset is good, and this patient made a complete recovery in 8 days.

Dissociative disorder frequently presents with neurological symptoms, and the commonest of these are convulsions, blindness, pain and amnesia. All of these symptoms will require full neurological investigation to exclude organic disease.

 KEY POINTS

- Dissociative disorder frequently presents as a neurological illness.
- The diagnosis of dissociative disorder must be one of exclusion.

CASE 19: UNSTEADINESS

History

A 32-year-old woman presents to the emergency department with unsteadiness of gait for 2 days. The problem has been more evident at night, but she feels a little unsteady on walking generally and on turning quickly. She had an upper respiratory infection a week or so earlier but has otherwise been well.

She smokes 10 cigarettes daily and drinks about 8–10 units of alcohol weekly. She has taken no recreational drugs. She is married with two children aged 2 and 6 years.

On systems review, there are no problems with appetite, bowels, micturition, menses or any other symptoms.

Two years previously, she had an episode of pain in the right eye associated with some blurring of vision in the right eye that lasted 2 to 3 weeks and then resolved spontaneously. She has had no subsequent visual problems. Her mother has type 2 diabetes mellitus.

Examination

She looks well. On neurological examination, she has nystagmus on lateral gaze in both eyes. There is a mild degree of incoordination on heel–shin testing in the left leg. She is unsteady on heel–toe walking, tending to fall to the left.

The blood pressure is 130/78 mmHg. On fundoscopy, there is pallor of the right optic disc.

🔍 INVESTIGATIONS

		Normal
Haemoglobin	14.5 g/dL	11.7–15.7 g/dL
Mean corpuscular volume (MCV)	88 fL	80–99 fL
White cell count	8.2×10^9/L	$3.5–11.0 \times 10^9$/L
Platelets	335×10^9/L	$150–440 \times 10^9$/L
Sodium	137 mmol/L	135–145 mmol/L
Potassium	4.3 mmol/L	3.5–5.0 mmol/L
Glucose	7.1 mmol/L	4.0–6.0 mmol/L
Urea	4.7 mmol/L	2.5–6.7 mmol/L
Creatinine	84 µmol/L	70–120 µmol/L

? QUESTIONS

- What is the most likely diagnosis?
- What further investigations would be appropriate?
- What management would be appropriate?

ANSWER 19

The findings of unsteadiness, nystagmus and incoordination all point to a cerebellar problem producing her gait disturbance. The only abnormal investigation is slightly raised blood glucose. She has a family history of diabetes and her blood glucose warrants further testing, but it is unlikely to be related to her current problem.

In the previous medical history, the episode of blurring of vision 2 years previously is characteristic of an episode of optic neuritis. Examination at the time would probably have shown a swollen pink optic nerve head. Residual changes may be the pale optic disc seen now, and detailed testing might show a residual visual problem. Optic neuritis is associated with recurrence and progression to further demyelinating problems in about 50% of cases (greater in women than men).

The combination of these two problems indicates two neurological problems separated in space and time, in typical sites for demyelination. This suggests a likely underlying diagnosis of multiple sclerosis (MS) according to the McDonald criteria.

Further investigations should be magnetic resonance imaging (MRI) to look for evidence of patchy demyelination. Abnormalities are found in the brain in more than 90% of patients and in the spinal cord in about 75%. Oedema is shown on T2-weighted images and cerebral atrophy and areas of axonal death on T1 images. If a lumbar puncture is performed, cerebrospinal fluid should be sent for oligoclonal bands and intrathecal IgG production. She also needs a detailed ophthalmological assessment. Other possible investigations are evoked potentials (visual, somatosensory or auditory) which may show subclinical lesions and help in the diagnosis by suggesting other areas of demyelination.

Immunomodulatory treatment with intravenous steroids, immunoglobulin or plasmapheresis may help in the initial episode and in affecting future progression. The monoclonal antibodies alemtuzumab (acts against T cells) and natalizumab (acts against VLA-4 receptors that allow immune cells to cross the blood–brain barrier) are now approved for relapsing and remitting disease. Disease modifying agents such as interferon beta help in relapsing cases of MS. Once the diagnosis is confirmed, she will need careful counselling around the question of possible future progression. She may benefit from contact with the MS Society UK.

 KEY POINTS

- Episodes of optic neuritis may be the first manifestation of MS.
- MRI is the optimal imaging technique for suspected MS.

CASE 20: HEADACHE

History

A 24-year-old man presents to an emergency department complaining of a severe, generalised headache, which started 24 hours previously and rapidly worsened. He has vomited twice and appears to be increasingly drowsy and confused. He finds bright lights uncomfortable. There is no significant medical history and he takes no regular medicines. There is no history of allergy. He smokes 10 cigarettes per day and drinks 24 units of alcohol per week. He is a graduate student doing an MA in psychology. He lives with his female partner, and they have two children, aged 3 and 4 years.

Examination

He looks flushed and unwell. His temperature is 39.2°C. He has stiffness on passive flexion of his neck. There is no rash. His sinuses are not tender and his eardrums appear normal. His pulse rate is 120/min, and blood pressure is 98/74 mmHg. Examination of heart, chest and abdomen is normal. His consciousness level is decreased, with a Glasgow Coma Scale (GCS) of 13/15, but he is rousable to command; there are no focal neurological signs. His fundi are normal, although examination is difficult due to photophobia.

🔍 INVESTIGATIONS

		Normal
Haemoglobin	13.9 g/dL	13.7–17.7 g/dL
White cell count	17.4 × 10⁹/L	3.9–10.6 × 10⁹/L
Platelets	322 × 10⁹/L	150–440 × 10⁹/L
Sodium	131 mmol/L	135–145 mmol/L
Potassium	3.9 mmol/L	3.5–5.0 mmol/L
Urea	10.4 mmol/L	2.5–6.7 mmol/L
Creatinine	176 µmol/L	70–120 µmol/L
Glucose	5.4 mmol/L	4.0–6.0 mmol/L
Blood cultures	results awaited	

Chest radiograph: normal

Electrocardiogram (ECG): sinus tachycardia

Computed tomography (CT) of brain: normal

Lumbar puncture	Turbid cerebrospinal fluid (CSF)	
Leucocytes	>8000/mL	<5/mL
CSF protein	1.4 g/L	<0.4 g/L
CSF glucose	0.8 mmol/L	>70% plasma glucose

Gram stain: result awaited

❓ QUESTIONS

- What is the diagnosis?
- What are the major differential diagnoses?
- How would you manage this patient?

DOI: 10.1201/9781003350934-22

ANSWER 20

This patient has bacterial meningitis. He has presented with sudden onset severe headache, vomiting, confusion, photophobia and neck stiffness. The presence of hypotension, neutrophilia and renal impairment suggests acute bacterial infection rather than viral infection. The triad of neck stiffness, fever and headache suggests meningitis as a differential. In patients in this age group, *Streptococcus pneumoniae* or *Neisseria meningitidis* are the most likely causative organisms. Rarely, Listeria can cause meningitis, and this is mostly in patients who are immunosuppressed (including patients who are elderly or pregnant).

Meningococcal meningitis (*N. meningitidis*) can be associated with a generalised vasculitic rash of meningococcal sepsis. The most severe headaches are experienced in meningitis, subarachnoid haemorrhage and classic migraine. Meningitis usually presents over hours, whereas subarachnoid haemorrhage usually presents suddenly. Other meningitis types include viral, fungal, cryptococcal and tuberculous meningitis, which can be distinguished by analysis of the CSF.

When meningitis is suspected, appropriate antibiotic treatment should be started even before the diagnosis is confirmed. In the absence of a history of significant penicillin allergy, the most common treatment would be intravenous ceftriaxone or cefotaxime, as these agents penetrate the CSF. Amoxicillin is added to patients who are over age 60, pregnant or immunocompromised due to the risk of Listeria. Dexamethasone is also recommended if within 12 hours after the first dose of antibiotics and continued if the meningitis is caused by pneumococcal meningitis.

Patients who are haemodynamically stable, with no papilloedema, seizures or lateralising neurological signs that suggest a space-occupying lesion, should have a lumbar puncture (LP) immediately. If there are localised neurological signs it is essential to perform a CT scan first to avoid the dangers of coning, which can occur when a LP is performed in the presence of raised intracranial pressure. If there is any delay in carrying out a CT head scan, antibiotics should be given prior to LP. The Gram stain and culture will give the definitive microbiological diagnosis which will help direct duration and type of antibiotic. In this case, the Gram stain demonstrated gram-positive diplococci consistent with *S. pneumoniae* infection.

Rapid initiation of intravenous antibiotics is essential. Adequate analgesia with opiates should be given. Fluid loss and hypotension should be treated with intravenous fluids and critical care teams should be involved early if hypotension is not responding to fluids.

His two children must be examined for signs of infection. If the causative organism was *N. meningitidis* or unknown, they should be given antibiotic prophylaxis and vaccinated against meningococcal meningitis. Meningococcal meningitis is a notifiable disease.

 KEY POINTS

- Bacterial meningitis causes severe headache, neck stiffness, drowsiness and photophobia.
- The main differential diagnoses are subarachnoid haemorrhage and migraine.
- LP is an essential investigation.
- If the patient has signs of severe infection, antibiotic treatment should be started before LP.

CASE 21: WEAKNESS

History

A 76-year-old woman presents to the emergency department complaining of an episode of weakness in her right arm and leg. She was sitting down with her husband when the weakness came on and her husband noticed that she slurred her speech. All of the symptoms resolved within 10 minutes. Her husband has noticed 2 to 3 episodes of slurred speech lasting a few minutes over the last 6 months but had thought nothing of it. Two months earlier, she had a sensation of darkness coming down over her left eye, lasting for a few minutes. She has had type 2 diabetes mellitus for 6 years, controlled on diet. She is hypertensive and suffered a myocardial infarction 3 years previously. She smokes about 10 cigarettes per day and drinks alcohol rarely. Her only medication is enalapril for her blood pressure.

Examination

She looks frail. Her pulse rate is 88/min and irregular and blood pressure is 172/94 mmHg. The apex beat is displaced to the sixth intercostal space, midaxillary line. Her heart sounds are normal, and a grade 3/6 pansystolic murmur is audible. A soft bruit is audible on auscultation over the left carotid artery. Her dorsalis pedis pulses are not palpable bilaterally, and her posterior tibial is weak on the left and absent on the right. Examination of her chest and abdomen is normal. Neurological examination demonstrates normal tone, power and reflexes. There is no sensory loss. Fundoscopy is normal.

INVESTIGATIONS		
		Normal
Haemoglobin	13.7 g/dL	11.7–15.7 g/dL
Mean corpuscular volume (MCV)	86 fL	80–99 fL
White cell count	7.4×10^9/L	$3.5–11.0 \times 10^9$/L
Platelets	242×10^9/L	$150–440 \times 10^9$/L
Sodium	137 mmol/L	135–145 mmol/L
Potassium	3.9 mmol/L	3.5–5.0 mmol/l
Urea	6.7 mmol/L	2.5–6.7 mmol/L
Creatinine	86 µmol/L	70–120 µmol/L
Glucose	5.8 mmol/L	4.0–6.0 mmol/L
Haemoglobin A_{1c} (HbA_{1c})	7.6%	<7%

Chest radiograph: normal

Electrocardiogram (ECG): atrial fibrillation

?	QUESTIONS

- What is the diagnosis?
- What investigations would you consider for this patient?
- How would you manage this patient?

DOI: 10.1201/9781003350934-23

ANSWER 21

This woman gives a history of transient neurological symptoms with no residual signs. She is at increased risk of cerebrovascular disease because of her smoking, hypertension and diabetes. She is describing recurrent transient ischaemic attacks (TIAs), which, by definition, resolve completely in less than 24 hours and, in practice, often much quicker. Two months before her admission, she had an episode of amaurosis fugax (transient uniocular blindness), which is often described to feel like a shutter coming down over the visual field of one eye. The TIAs affect the left cerebral hemisphere area of the brain supplied by the left carotid artery, causing right-sided weakness and dysarthria. TIAs may be caused by thromboembolisms from ulcerated plaques in the carotid arteries or aortic arch, from cardiac sources such as a dilated left atrium and, more rarely, due to haematological causes such as polycythaemia rubra vera, sickle cell disease or hyperviscosity due to myeloma. The symptoms may be the same each time or vary. Her ECG shows atrial fibrillation, and she has signs of mitral regurgitation with a pansystolic murmur and displaced apex beat. There are three obvious potential sources for emboli:

- A left carotid artery stenosis (in a correct location to account for the distribution of these TIAs and more likely in the presence of a carotid bruit).
- The left atrium in atrial fibrillation with clinically evident mitral regurgitation.
- A previous myocardial infarction with mural thrombosis.

!   MAJOR CAUSES OF TRANSIENT NEUROLOGICAL SYNDROMES

- **Migraine:** The aura of migraine is a spreading and slowly intensifying phenomenon, and the symptoms are usually positive (e.g., scotomata). The aura is usually followed by a severe headache. However, migraines can be associated with focal neurological deficits (e.g., hemiplegia).
- **Focal epilepsy:** This also normally causes positive symptoms such as twitching and sensory symptoms, which may march up one limb and from one limb to another on the same side.
- **Syncope:** Unlike most TIAs, there is loss of consciousness, but there are usually no focal signs. Dizziness often precedes the attack.
- **Space-occupying lesion:** A cerebral tumour or abscess can produce fluctuating symptoms and signs. The symptoms are usually more gradual in onset and are often associated with headaches or personality changes.
- **Miscellaneous:** Hysteria, cervical spondylosis, hypoglycaemia and cataplexy.

This patient should be investigated with computed tomography (CT) of the head to exclude a structural space-occupying lesion; echocardiography to assess left-atrial size, the mitral valve (to exclude infective valvular vegetations) and to rule out thrombus in the left ventricle related to the previous infarct; and a Doppler ultrasound of the carotid arteries. If a critical carotid stenosis (>70%) is present, carotid endarterectomy should be considered. The patient should be anticoagulated with warfarin because of her atrial fibrillation and carotid stenosis. Her blood pressure and diabetes should be carefully controlled and her lipids measured and treated if appropriate.

🔑 KEY POINTS

- Most transient ischaemic attacks persist for only a few minutes.
- Approximately 40% of patients with cerebral infarction have a prior history of TIAs.
- Multiple risk factors need to be considered in the investigation and management of vascular disease.

CASE 22: WEAKNESS OF THE LEGS

History

A 48-year-old man presents to the emergency department with weakness of his legs. Four days before admission, he had pins and needles in his feet and 3 days before admission, he developed difficulty walking, which progressed to difficulty standing. His bowel and bladder are functioning normally. He has no significant medical history, though does report a brief episode of gastro-enteritis 4 weeks prior to onset of symptoms. He neither smokes nor drinks alcohol and is taking no medication. He works in a local supermarket.

Examination

He looks well but is anxious. His pulse rate is 102/min and blood pressure is 152/94 mmHg. His jugular venous pressure is not raised, and examination of his heart, respiratory and abdominal systems is otherwise normal. Neurological examination shows MRC grade 2/5 power below his knees and 3/5 power for hip flexion/extension. The tone in his legs is reduced. Knee and ankle reflex are absent even with reinforcement. There is impaired pinprick sensation up to the knees and reduced joint position sense and vibration sense in the ankles. Neurological examination of his arms is normal.

 INVESTIGATIONS

Initial haematology and biochemistry results are normal.
A lumbar puncture is performed with the following results:

		Normal
Cerebrospinal fluid (CSF): clear		
Pressure	170 mm CSF	<200 mm CSF
CSF protein	3.4 g/L	<0.4 g/L
CSF glucose	4 mmol/L	>70% plasma glucose
Leucocytes	5/mL	<5/mL
Plasma glucose	4.5 mmol/L	4.0–6.0 mmol/L

Gram stain: no organisms

? QUESTIONS

- What is the diagnosis?
- What are the major differential diagnoses?
- How would you manage this patient?

DOI: 10.1201/9781003350934-24

ANSWER 22

The most marked feature is the loss of power. The reduced tone and absent reflexes indicate that this is a lower motor neurone lesion. The sensory disturbance is less severe, and he has a sensory level around L/3. This is the typical clinical picture of Guillain–Barré syndrome (acute idiopathic inflammatory polyneuropathy). This disorder is a polyneuropathy that develops usually over 2–3 weeks, but sometimes more rapidly. It most commonly follows *Campylobacter* gastroenteritis or a viral infection such as influenza, cytomegalovirus or human immunodeficiency virus, and a fever is common. It predominantly causes motor neuropathy, which can have a proximal, distal or generalised distribution. Distal paraesthesia and sensory loss are common. Reflexes are lost early. Cranial and bulbar nerve paralysis may occur and respiratory muscle involvement can cause respiratory failure. The diagnosis is made from the clinical picture and can be confirmed with examination of the CSF and from nerve conduction studies. The CSF protein is usually raised, but the cell count is usually normal, although there may be mild lymphocytosis. The disorder is probably due to a cell-mediated delayed hypersensitivity reaction causing myelin to be stripped off the axons by mononuclear cells.

> **!   DIFFERENTIAL DIAGNOSES OF MOTOR NEUROPATHY**
>
> - Guillain–Barré syndrome
> - Lead poisoning
> - Diphtheria
> - Charcot–Marie–Tooth disease (hereditary motor and sensory neuropathy)
> - Poliomyelitis

An acute-onset neuropathy suggests:

- Guillain–Barré syndrome
- Porphyria
- Malignancy
- Some toxic neuropathies
- Diphtheria
- Botulism

This patient should be referred to a neurologist for further investigation and management. In any patient who presents with weakness and sensory signs, it is important to make sure there is no evidence of spinal cord compression or multiple sclerosis. These may acutely present with hypotonia. However, eventually they tend to cause hypertonia, hyper-reflexia and a more distinct sensory level. His respiratory function should be monitored with daily bedside spirometry, and temporary non-invasive ventilator support or intubation may be necessary. Supportive care is the most important element of treatment. He should also be treated with either plasma exchange or intravenous immunoglobulin (IVIG), which will hasten recovery. Most patients recover over a period of several weeks.

> **🔑   KEY POINTS**
>
> - Guillain–Barré syndrome presents with predominantly a motor neuropathy, although sensory symptoms are usually present.
> - Management involves close monitoring of forced vital capacity (FVC), rapid respiratory support if needed and consideration of IVIG.
> - There is often a history of an infective illness in the previous 3 weeks, often *Campylobacter jejuni*.

CASE 23: CLUMSINESS

History

A 66-year-old woman notices that she is having trouble performing some everyday tasks, such as doing up buttons on her blouse and chopping vegetables for cooking. She complains that her muscles feel stiff, and it is taking her longer than it did to walk to the local shops. She is anxious about these problems since she lives alone and has to do everything for herself. She has noticed a little shakiness, which she ascribes to anxiety. Her daughter has told her that it is becoming increasingly difficult to read the small writing in the letters she sends. She is a retired journalist and has no significant past medical history. There is no disturbance of her bowels or micturition. Her appetite has been good and her weight steady. She complains that she has been sleeping poorly and is consequently rather tired. She does not smoke tobacco and drinks only occasionally. She has hypertension and takes 50 mg atenolol daily.

Examination

Her pulse is 60/min and regular and her blood pressure is 134/84 mmHg. There are no abnormalities in the cardiovascular or respiratory systems. On neurological examination, there is no muscle wasting. She has generally increased muscle tone throughout the range of movement, equal in flexors and extensors. There is a slight tremor affecting mainly her right hand, which is suppressed when she tries to do something. She has problems with fine tasks such as doing up buttons. Power, reflexes, coordination and sensation are all normal. When asked to walk, she is a little slow to get started and has difficulty stopping and turning.

? | **QUESTIONS**

- What is the diagnosis?
- How would you investigate this patient?
- How would you manage this patient?

ANSWER 23

There is evidence in the history and examination of tremor, rigidity and bradykinesia. Her writing shows micrographia secondary to the rigidity and slowness of movement. Her hypertension is well controlled on the beta-blocker. Beta-blockers can cause tiredness and slowness but not to the extent seen in this woman. This woman has Parkinson's disease, presenting with the classic extrapyramidal triad of tremor, rigidity and hypokinesia. Tremor is usually an early symptom and may be unilateral. The combination of tremor with rigidity leads to the cogwheel form of rigidity. The patient often goes on to have a blank mask-like facies. There is difficulty starting to walk (freezing), and the patient uses small steps and has difficulty stopping (festination). There is generally normal intellectual function, but there is often depression. Sleep is often disturbed, contributing to daytime tiredness. The characteristic pathological abnormality is degeneration of dopamine-secreting neurones in the nigrostriatal pathway of the basal ganglia.

Parkinsonian features (parkinsonism) may occur in a variety of diseases:

- Parkinson's disease
- Postencephalitic parkinsonism
- Neuroleptic drug-induced Parkinson's disease
- Parkinsonism in association with Alzheimer's/multi-infarct dementia

---

! | **CLASSIFICATION OF TREMOR**

- **Rest tremor:** The tremor is worse at rest and is typical of parkinsonism.
- **Postural tremor:** This is characteristic of benign essential tremor, physiological tremor and exaggerated physiological tremor caused by anxiety, alcohol and thyrotoxicosis. Benign essential tremor is not present at rest, but appears on holding the arms outstretched, but is not worse on movement (finger–nose testing). Tests of coordination are normal and walking is unaffected. There is usually a family history of tremor, and the tremor is helped by alcohol and beta-blockers.
- **Intention tremor:** The tremor is worse on movement and is most obvious in finger–nose testing. It is usually caused by brainstem or cerebellar disease caused by such diseases as multiple sclerosis, localised tumours or spinocerebellar degeneration.

A variety of drugs are available to treat this patient's Parkinson's disease. During early disease, dopaminergic supplementation often sufficiently reduces or eliminates symptoms. Levodopa is the preferred initial treatment, used in combination with carbidopa, a selective dopa decarboxylase inhibitor which does not cross the blood–brain barrier, reducing peripheral adverse effects. The commonest side effects are nausea, vomiting, dizziness, postural hypotension and neuropsychiatric problems. After many years of treatment, the effects tend to diminish and the patient may develop rapid oscillations in control—the 'on–off' effect. When these develop, a sustained-release formulation of levodopa or a dopamine agonist may produce improvement. Amantadine may also be useful in reducing dyskinesias that occur with dopamine medication. Some clinicians may delay starting treatment due to its loss of effect over time. This requires careful discussion with the individual patient. Deep brain stimulation may be considered for refractory complications in patients with moderate to severe Parkinson's. Exercise should always be encouraged, as this has been shown to improve functional performance on motor tasks at any stage of disease. She should be assessed by a physiotherapist, occupational therapist and speech therapist and provided with advice and aids. With time, her house may need to be altered to aid her mobility.

 KEY POINTS

- Parkinson's disease is characterised by tremor, rigidity and hypokinesia.
- Patient management is long term and multidisciplinary.
- Benefits of levodopa treatment in Parkinson's disease may lessen with time.

Section 3
RHEUMATOLOGY

CASE 24: PAINFUL KNEE

History

A 35-year-old man is seen in the emergency department because he has developed a painful, swollen right knee. This has occurred rapidly over the past 36 hours. There is no history of trauma to the knee or previous joint problems. He feels generally unwell and has also noticed his eyes are sore. He has had no significant previous medical illnesses. He is married with two children. He is a non-smoker and drinks about 15 units of alcohol per week. He is a businessman and returned 3 weeks ago from a business trip to Thailand.

Examination

His temperature is 38.0°C. Both eyes appear red. There is a brown macular rash on his palms and soles. Examination of cardiovascular, respiratory, abdominal and neurological systems is normal. His right knee is swollen, hot and tender with limitation in flexion. No other joint appears to be affected.

🔍 INVESTIGATIONS

		Normal
Haemoglobin	13.8 g/dL	13.3–17.7 g/dL
Mean corpuscular volume (MCV)	87 fL	80–99 fL
White cell count	13.6×10^9/L	$3.9–10.6 \times 10^9$/L
Platelets	345×10^9/L	$150–440 \times 10^9$/L
Erythrocyte sedimentation rate (ESR)	64 mm/h	<10 mm/h
Sodium	139 mmol/L	135–145 mmol/L
Potassium	4.1 mmol/L	3.5–5.0 mmol/L
Urea	5.2 mmol/L	2.5–6.7 mmol/L
Creatinine	94 µmol/L	70–120 µmol/L

Urinalysis: no protein; no blood; no glucose
Blood cultures: negative
Radiograph of the knee: soft-tissue swelling around joint

❓ QUESTIONS

- What are the major differential diagnoses?
- What is the diagnosis?
- How would you investigate and manage this patient?

ANSWER 24

This patient has a monoarthropathy, a rash and red eyes. Investigations show a raised white cell count and ESR. The diagnosis in this man is post-infective inflammatory mucositis and arthritis, often shortened to reactive arthritis. This disease classically presents with a triad of symptoms (although all three may not always be present):

- Seronegative arthritis affecting mainly lower limb joints
- Conjunctivitis
- Non-specific urethritis (NSU)

The trigger can be non-gonococcal urethritis (*Chlamydia trachomatis*) or certain enteric infections (*Salmonella*, *Shigella*, *Yersinia* and *Campylobacter.*) This patient is likely to have contracted NSU after sexual intercourse in Thailand. On direct questioning, he admitted to the presence of urethral discharge. The acute arthritis is typically a monoarthritis but can develop into a chronic relapsing destructive arthritis affecting the knees and feet and cause sacroiliitis and spondylitis. Tendonitis and plantar fasciitis may occur. The red eyes are due to conjunctivitis and anterior uveitis and can recur with flares of the arthritis. The rash on the patient's palmar surfaces is the characteristic brown macular rash of this condition: keratoderma blennorrhagica. Other features of this condition include nail dystrophy and a circinate balanitis. Systemic manifestations such as pericarditis, pleuritis, fever and lymphadenopathy may occur in this disease. The ESR is usually elevated.

! DIFFERENTIAL DIAGNOSES OF AN ACUTE MONOARTHRITIS

- **Gonococcal arthritis:** Occasionally a polyarthritis affecting the small joints of the hands and wrists, with a pustular rash.
- **Acute septic arthritis:** The patient looks ill and septic, and the skin over the joint is very erythematous.
- **Other seronegative arthritides:** Ankylosing spondylitis, psoriatic arthropathy.
- **Viral arthritis:** Usually polyarticular.
- **Acute rheumatoid arthritis:** Usually polyarticular.
- **Acute gout:** Most commonly affects the metatarsophalangeal joints.
- **Pseudogout:** Caused by sodium pyrophosphate crystals; often affects large joints in older patients.
- **Lyme disease:** Caused by *Borrelia burgdorferi* infection transmitted by a tick bite; may have the characteristic skin rash erythema migrans.
- **Haemorrhagic arthritis:** Usually a history of trauma or bleeding disorder.

This patient should have urethral swabs taken to exclude chlamydial/gonococcal infections and the appropriate antibiotics given. His knee should be aspirated. A Gram stain will exclude a pyogenic infection and birefringent microscopy can be used to detect uric acid or pyrophosphate crystals. This patient should be given non-steroidal anti-inflammatory drugs (NSAIDs) for the pain, and he may require intra-articular steroids or oral prednisolone.

🔑 KEY POINTS

- The most likely causes of an acute large joint monoarthritis are septic arthritis and seronegative arthritis.
- Septic arthritis must be recognised and treated as a medical emergency as it can cause rapid destruction of the joint and septicaemia.

CASE 25: PAIN IN THE KNEE

History

An 80-year-old woman presents to her general practitioner (GP) with pain and swelling in her left knee. The pain began 2 days previously and she says that the knee is now hot, swollen and painful on movement. In the past, she has a history of mild osteoarthritis of the hips. She has occasional heartburn and indigestion. She had a health check 6 months previously and was told that everything was fine except for some elevation of her blood pressure, which was 172/102 mmHg and her creatinine level, which was around the upper limit of normal. The blood pressure was checked several times over the next 4 weeks and found to be persistently elevated and she was started on treatment with 2.5 mg bendroflumethiazide. The last blood pressure reading was 148/84 mmHg. There is no relevant family history. She has never smoked and her alcohol consumption averages 4 units per week. She takes occasional paracetamol for hip pain.

Examination

Her blood pressure is 142/86 mmHg. The temperature is 37.5°C and the pulse is 88/min. There is grade 2 hypertensive retinopathy. There is no other abnormality on cardiovascular or respiratory examination. In the hands, there are Heberden's nodes over the distal interphalangeal joints.

The left knee is hot and swollen with evidence of effusion in the joint with a positive patellar tap. There is pain on flexion beyond 90 degrees. The right knee appears normal.

🔍 INVESTIGATIONS

		Normal
Haemoglobin	12.1 g/dL	11.7–15.7 g/dL
White cell count	12.4 × 10⁹/L	3.5–11.0 × 10⁹/L
Platelets	384 × 10⁹/L	150–440 × 10⁹/L
Erythrocyte sedimentation rate (ESR)	48 mm/h	<10 mm/h
Sodium	136 mmol/L	135–145 mmol/L
Potassium	3.6 mmol/L	3.5–5.0 mmol/L
Urea	7.3 mmol/L	2.5–6.7 mmol/L
Creatinine	116 μmol/L	70–120 μmol/L
Glucose	10.8 mmol/L	4.0–6.0 mmol/L

A radiograph of the knees is performed, and the result is shown in Figure 25.1.

DOI: 10.1201/9781003350934-28

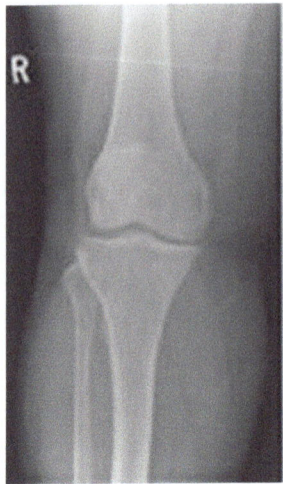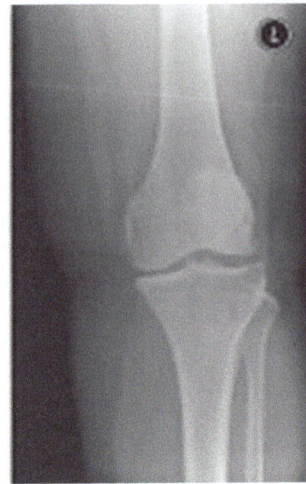

Figure 25.1 Radiograph of both knees.

? | **QUESTIONS**

- What is your interpretation of the findings?
- What is the likely diagnosis?
- What is the appropriate management?

ANSWER 25

The clinical picture is one of an acute monoarthritis. The patient has a history of some hip pains, but this and the Heberden's nodes are common findings in an 80-year-old woman, related to osteoarthritis. The blood results show a raised white cell count and ESR, a raised blood sugar and renal function at the upper limit of normal.

> **!**   **DIFFERENTIAL DIAGNOSES OF PAIN IN THE KNEE**
>
> The differential diagnosis includes:
> * Trauma
> * Septic arthritis
> * Gout
> * Pseudogout

The recent introduction of a thiazide diuretic for treatment of hypertension increases the suspicion of gout. Pseudogout is caused by deposition of calcium pyrophosphate crystals and would be expected to show calcification in the articular cartilage in the knee joint. The radiographs here show some joint space narrowing but no evidence of calcification in the articular cartilage. The fever, high white cell count and ESR are compatible with acute gout. The raised glucose may also be a side effect of thiazide diuretics. If this remains after the acute arthritis has subsided, then it may need further treatment. Precipitation of gout by thiazides is more likely in older women, particularly in the presence of renal impairment and diabetes. It may involve the hands, be polyarticular, and can affect existing Heberden's nodes.

The serum uric acid level is likely to be raised, but this occurs commonly without evidence of acute gout. The definitive investigation is aspiration of the joint. The fluid should be sent for culture and inspection with a specific request for inspection for crystals. A high white cell count would be expected in an acute inflammatory arthritis. The diagnosis is made from the needle-like crystals of uric acid, which are negatively birefringent under polarised light, unlike the positively birefringent crystals of calcium pyrophosphate.

In this case, the pain in the joint was partly relieved by the aspiration. Treatment with a non-steroidal anti-inflammatory drug should be covered by a proton pump inhibitor in view of her history of heartburn and indigestion. The thiazide diuretic was changed to an angiotensin-converting enzyme inhibitor as treatment for her hypertension, and the blood glucose elevation resolved. A short course of prednisolone can also be used in acute gout. A xanthine oxidase inhibitor such as allopurinol might be considered if the serum urate remained raised or the condition did not settle after stopping the thiazide diuretic.

>   **KEY POINTS**
>
> * A careful drug history is an essential part of the history.
> * Thiazide diuretics can precipitate diabetes and gout, especially in the elderly.

CASE 26: JOINT PAINS

History

A 38-year-old woman presents to her general practitioner (GP) complaining of pains in her joints. She has noticed these pains worsening over several months. Her joints are most stiff on waking in the mornings. The joints that are most painful are the small joints of the hands and feet. The pain is relieved by diclofenac tablets. She feels tired and has lost 4 kg in weight over 3 months. She has had no previous serious illnesses. She is married with two children and works as a legal secretary. She is a non-smoker and drinks alcohol only occasionally. Her only medication is diclofenac.

Examination

On examination, she looks pale and is clinically anaemic. Her proximal interphalangeal joints and metacarpophalangeal joints are swollen and painful, with effusions present. Her metatarsophalangeal joints are also tender. Physical examination is otherwise normal.

<table>
<tr><td>🔍</td><td colspan="3">INVESTIGATIONS</td></tr>
<tr><td></td><td></td><td></td><td>Normal</td></tr>
<tr><td></td><td>Haemoglobin</td><td>8.9 g/dL</td><td>11.7–15.7 g/dL</td></tr>
<tr><td></td><td>Mean corpuscular volume (MCV)</td><td>87 fL</td><td>80–99 fL</td></tr>
<tr><td></td><td>White cell count</td><td>7.2×10^9/L</td><td>$3.5–11.0 \times 10^9$/L</td></tr>
<tr><td></td><td>Platelets</td><td>438×10^9/L</td><td>$150–440 \times 10^9$/l</td></tr>
<tr><td></td><td>Erythrocyte sedimentation rate (ESR)</td><td>78 mm/h</td><td><10 mm/h</td></tr>
<tr><td></td><td>Sodium</td><td>141 mmol/L</td><td>135–145 mmol/L</td></tr>
<tr><td></td><td>Potassium</td><td>3.9 mmol/L</td><td>3.5–5.0 mmol/L</td></tr>
<tr><td></td><td>Urea</td><td>6.9 mmol/L</td><td>2.5–6.7 mmol/L</td></tr>
<tr><td></td><td>Creatinine</td><td>125 µmol/L</td><td>70–120 µmol/L</td></tr>
<tr><td></td><td>Glucose</td><td>4.6 mmol/L</td><td>4.0–6.0 mmol/L</td></tr>
<tr><td></td><td>Albumin</td><td>33 g/L</td><td>35–50 g/L</td></tr>
</table>

Urinalysis: no protein; no blood; no glucose

? QUESTIONS

- What is the diagnosis and what are the major differential diagnoses?
- How would you investigate this patient?
- How would you manage this patient?

ANSWER 26

This patient has symptoms and signs typical of early rheumatoid arthritis. Rheumatoid arthritis is a chronic, systemic inflammatory disorder principally affecting joints in a peripheral symmetrical distribution. The peak incidence is between 35 and 55 years in women and 40 and 60 years in men. It is a disease with a long course with exacerbations and remissions. The acute presentation may occur over the course of a day and be associated with fever and malaise. More commonly, as in this case, it presents insidiously and this group has a worse prognosis. Rheumatoid arthritis characteristically affects proximal interphalangeal, metacarpophalangeal and wrist joints in the hands and metatarsophalangeal joints, ankles, knees and cervical spine.

Early morning stiffness of the joints is typical of rheumatoid arthritis. As the disease progresses, damage to cartilage, bone and tendons leads to the characteristic deformities of this condition. Extra-articular features include rheumatoid nodules, vasculitis causing cutaneous nodules and digital gangrene, scleritis, pleural effusions, diffuse pulmonary fibrosis, pulmonary nodules, obliterative bronchiolitis, pericarditis and splenomegaly (Felty's syndrome). There is usually a normochromic, normocytic anaemia and raised ESR, as seen here. The degree of anaemia and ESR roughly correlates with disease activity. In this case, the raised creatinine is probably due to the use of diclofenac. Non-steroidal anti-inflammatory drugs (NSAIDs) reduce the glomerular filtration rate in all patients. Rarely, they can cause an acute interstitial nephritis. In patients with long-standing rheumatoid arthritis, renal infiltration by amyloid may occur.

! DIFFERENTIAL DIAGNOSIS OF AN ACUTE SYMMETRICAL POLYARTHRITIS

- **Osteoarthritis:** Characteristically affects the distal interphalangeal as well as proximal interphalangeal and first metacarpophalangeal joints.
- **Rheumatoid arthritis:** Characteristically affects proximal interphalangeal, metacarpophalangeal and wrist joints in the hands.
- **Systemic lupus erythematosus:** Usually causes a mild, flitting, non-erosive arthritis.
- **Gout:** usually starts as monoarthritis.
- **Seronegative arthritides:** Ankylosing spondylitis, psoriasis, Reiter's disease. These usually cause asymmetrical arthritis, affecting medium and larger joints as well as the sacroiliac and distal interphalangeal joints.
- **Acute viral arthritis (e.g., rubella):** Resolves completely.

This patient should be referred to a rheumatologist for further investigation and management. The affected joints should be radiographed. If there has been joint damage, the radiograph will show subluxation, juxta-articular osteoporosis, loss of joint space and bony erosions. A common site for erosions to be found in early rheumatoid arthritis is the fifth metatarsophalangeal joint (arrowed in Figure 26.1). Blood tests should be taken for rheumatoid factor (present in rheumatoid arthritis) and anti-DNA antibodies (present in systemic lupus erythematosus). This patient should be given NSAIDs for analgesia and to reduce joint stiffness to allow her to continue her secretarial work. Disease-modifying drugs such as hydroxychloroquine, sulfasalazine, methotrexate or leflunomide should be considered unless the patient settles easily on NSAIDs. Addition of an anti-tumour necrosis factor (TNF) antibody is considered where the disease fails to come under control with methotrexate.

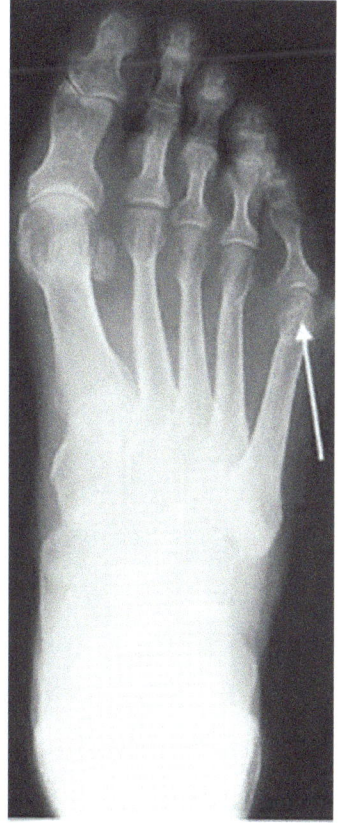

Figure 26.1 Radiograph of the foot.

🔑   **KEY POINTS**

- Rheumatoid arthritis tends to spare the distal interphalangeal joints.
- Systemic symptoms of rheumatoid arthritis may precede the joint symptoms.
- Anaemia and ESR correlate with disease activity.
- NSAIDs may adversely affect renal function.

History

A 75-year-old woman presents to her general practitioner (GP) complaining of severe back pain. This developed suddenly a week previously after carrying a heavy suitcase at the airport. The pain is persistent and in her lower back. She has had increasing problems with back pain over the past 10 years and her family has commented on how stooped her posture has become. Her height has decreased by about 10 cm over this period. Her past medical history is notable for severe chronic asthma. She takes courses of oral corticosteroids often for several months three to four times a year and uses steroid inhalers on a regular basis. She fell 2 years ago and sustained a Colles' fracture to her left wrist. Her menopause occurred at 42 years. She smokes 30 cigarettes a day and drinks 4 bottles of wine a week.

Examination

She has thoracic kyphosis. She is tender over the L4 vertebra. She has some abdominal striae and a number of bruises on her arms and thighs. She is not anaemic and examination is otherwise unremarkable.

🔍 INVESTIGATIONS

		Normal
Haemoglobin	11.9 g/dL	11.7–15.7 g/dL
Mean corpuscular volume (MCV)	103 fL	80–99 fL
White cell count	6.2×10^9/L	$3.5–11.0 \times 10^9$/L
Platelets	358×10^9/L	$150–440 \times 10^9$/L
Erythrocyte sedimentation rate (ESR)	8 mm/h	<10 mm/h
Sodium	143 mmol/L	135–145 mmol/L
Potassium	4.9 mmol/L	3.5–5.0 mmol/L
Urea	5.9 mmol/L	2.5–6.7 mmol/L
Creatinine	102 µmol/L	70–120 µmol/L
Calcium	2.42 mmol/L	2.12–2.65 mmol/L
Phosphate	1.26 mmol/L	0.8–1.45 mmol/L
Alkaline phosphatase	156 IU/L	30–300 IU/L

The radiograph of the lumbar spine is shown in Figure 27.1.

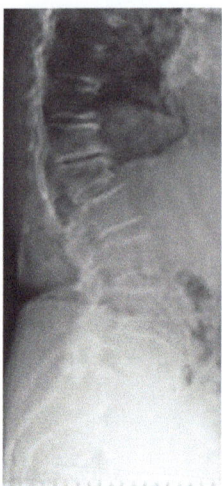

Figure 27.1 Radiograph of the lumbar spine.

? | QUESTIONS

- What is your interpretation of the findings?
- What is the likely diagnosis?
- How would you manage this patient?

ANSWER 27

This woman has a kyphosis, localised back pain and radiological evidence of fracture, indicating a likely diagnosis of vertebral collapse secondary to osteoporosis. The loss of height is typical and is usually noted more by others than the patient. The back pain is due to collapse of the vertebrae. This can occur spontaneously or in association with a recognised stress, such as lifting or carrying a heavy load. Examination confirms loss of trunk height, thoracic kyphosis and proximity of the ribs to the iliac crest.

> **! DIFFERENTIAL DIAGNOSES OF OSTEOPOROSIS**
>
> - Multiple myeloma
> - Metastatic carcinoma, particularly from the prostate, breast, bronchus, thyroid and kidney
> - Osteomalacia
> - Hyperparathyroidism
> - Steroid therapy or Cushing's syndrome

This patient has several risk factors for osteoporosis. First, she is 75 years old and ageing is associated with bone loss. Second, she has been postmenopausal for more than 30 years. Premenopausal ovarian production of oestrogens helps to preserve bone mass. Third, she has been on oral and inhaled corticosteroids for her asthma for years. Finally, excess alcohol intake may also be a factor. Her red cells are macrocytic, which is consistent with heavy alcohol intake. Alcohol can lead to an increased incidence of falls and fractures. She has no clinical evidence of thyrotoxicosis or hypopituitarism, which can cause osteoporosis.

This woman should have blood tests to exclude myeloma, cancer and metabolic bone disease. Patients with myeloma are typically anaemic with a raised ESR and a monoclonal paraprotein band on serum protein electrophoresis. In contrast to metabolic bone diseases, biochemical measurements (serum calcium, alkaline phosphatase and parathormone [PTH]) in osteoporosis are normal. She should have plain radiographs of her spine. Collapse of the vertebral body will manifest as irregular anterior wedging affecting some vertebrae and not others (L1 and L4). A dual-energy X-ray absorptiometry (DEXA) scan can be performed to assess the severity of the osteoporosis, but treatment is indicated anyway with a fracture at this age.

She should have her dose of corticosteroids reduced to the minimum required to control her asthmatic symptoms, using the inhaled routes as much as possible. Inhaled steroids can cause bruising and systemic effects in prolonged high dose but rarely cause osteoporosis and are considerably safer than oral corticosteroids. She should be started on calcium and vitamin D supplements and a bisphosphonate to try to reduce her bone loss. Oestrogen-based hormone replacement therapy is only used for symptoms associated with menopause because of the increased incidence of thromboembolism and endometrial carcinoma. Other possible treatments for osteoporosis include denosumab, which reduces the activity of osteoclasts, therefore reducing the breakdown of bone.

>   **KEY POINTS**
>
> - Osteoporosis is common in the elderly.
> - Bone loss is more rapid in post-menopausal women than men.
> - DEXA scan is the method of choice for screening for osteoporosis.
> - There are increasingly effective treatments available for the treatment of osteoporosis.

CASE 28: UNCONSCIOUS AT HOME

History

A 28-year-old woman is admitted to the emergency department in a coma. The patient was found unconscious on the floor by her boyfriend. She had not been seen by anyone for the previous 48 hours. No history was available from the patient, but her partner volunteered the information that they are both intravenous heroin addicts. She is unemployed, smokes 25 cigarettes per day, drinks 40 units of alcohol per week and has used heroin for the past 4 years. They have occasionally shared needles with other addicts. They both had negative human immunodeficiency virus (HIV) tests about 1 year ago. She has not made any suicide attempts in the past. She has had no other medical illnesses. She has lost touch with her family.

Examination

There are multiple old, scarred needle puncture sites. Her pulse is 64/min and regular, blood pressure is 110/60 mmHg, jugular venous pressure is not raised and heart sounds are normal. Her respiratory rate is 12/min and she has dullness to percussion and bronchial breathing at the left base posteriorly. Abdominal examination is normal. Her consciousness level is depressed but she is rousable to painful stimuli. She has pinpoint pupils but has no focal neurological signs. A bolus injection of intravenous naloxone causes her conscious level to rise transiently. Her left arm is swollen and painful from the shoulder down.

DOI: 10.1201/9781003350934-31

🔍 INVESTIGATIONS		
		Normal
Haemoglobin	13.6 g/dL	13.3–17.7 g/dL
White cell count	9.2 × 10⁹/L	3.9–10.6 × 10⁹/L
Platelets	233 × 10⁹/L	150–440 × 10⁹/L
Sodium	137 mmol/L	135–145 mmol/L
Potassium	7.8 mmol/L	3.5–5.0 mmol/L
Urea	42.3 mmol/L	2.5–6.7 mmol/L
Creatinine	622 µmol/L	70–120 µmol/L
Bicarbonate	14 mmol/L	24–30 mmol/L
Glucose	4.1 mmol/L	4.0–6.0 mmol/L
Calcium	1.64 mmol/L	2.12–2.65 mmol/L
Phosphate	3.6 mmol/L	0.8–1.45 mmol/L
Creatine kinase	68,000 IU/L	25–195 IU/L
Arterial blood gases on air		
pH	7.27	7.38–7.44
pco₂	7.5 kPa	4.7–6.0 kPa
po₂	9.2 kPa	12.0–14.5 kPa

Urinalysis: + protein; +++ blood. Urine microscopy: brown urine; no red cells; many granular casts. Electrocardiogram (ECG): flattened P-wave; peaked T-waves. Chest radiograph: extensive left-lower-zone consolidation.

? QUESTIONS
• What is the cause of this patient's acute renal failure?
• What further immediate and treatment does this woman need?
• What management needs to be considered in the long term?

ANSWER 28

This patient has acute renal failure as a result of rhabdomyolysis. Severe muscle damage causes a massively elevated serum creatine kinase (CK) level and a rise in serum potassium and phosphate levels. In this case, she has laid unconscious on her left arm for many hours due to an overdose of alcohol and intravenous heroin. As a result, she has developed severe ischaemic muscle damage, causing release of myoglobin, which is toxic to the kidneys. Other causes of rhabdomyolysis include crush injuries, severe hypokalaemia, excessive exercise, myopathies, drugs (e.g., ciclosporin and statins) and certain viral infections. The urine is dark because of the presence of myoglobin, which causes a false-positive dipstick test for blood. Myoglobin has a half-life of 2–3 hours much shorter than CK, thus, myoglobinuria has often disappeared whilst the CK is still raised.

Acute renal failure due to rhabdomyolysis causes profound hypocalcaemia in the oliguric phase due to calcium sequestration in muscle and reduced 1,25-dihydroxycalciferol levels, often with rebound hypercalcaemia in the recovery phase. This woman's consciousness level is still depressed as a result of opiate and alcohol toxicity and she has clinical and radiological evidence of aspiration pneumonia. She has mixed metabolic and respiratory acidosis (low pH, bicarbonate) due to acute renal failure and respiratory depression (pCO_2 elevated). Her arterial oxygenation is reduced due to hypoventilation and pneumonia. She also has compartment syndrome in her arm due to massive swelling of her damaged muscles.

This patient has life-threatening hyperkalaemia with electrocardiogram (ECG) changes. The ECG changes of hyperkalaemia progress from the earliest signs of peaking of the T-wave, P-wave flattening, prolongation of the PR interval through to widening of the QRS complex, a sine-wave pattern and ventricular fibrillation. Emergency treatment involves intravenous calcium gluconate, which stabilises cardiac conduction and intravenous insulin/glucose, intravenous sodium bicarbonate and nebulised salbutamol, all of which temporarily lower the plasma potassium by increasing the cellular uptake of potassium. However, these steps should be regarded as holding measures while urgent dialysis is being organised.

The chest radiograph and clinical findings indicate consolidation of the left lower lobe. This patient should initially be managed on an intensive care unit. She will require antibiotics for her pneumonia and will require a naloxone infusion or mechanical ventilation for her respiratory failure. The patient should have vigorous rehydration with monitoring of her central venous pressure. If a good urinary flow can be maintained, urinary pH should be kept greater than 7.0 by bicarbonate infusion, which prevents the renal toxicity of myoglobin. This patient also needs to be considered urgently for surgical fasciotomy to relieve the compartment syndrome in her arm.

In the longer term, the patient needs counselling and, with her boyfriend, should be offered access to drug rehabilitation services. They should also be offered testing for blood-borne viruses (hepatitis B and C and human immunodeficiency virus [HIV]).

🔑 **KEY POINTS**

- A very high creatine kinase level is diagnostic of rhabdomyolysis. The red/brown urine of myoglobinuria may be absent at presentation because of the speed of clearance of myoglobin.
- As statins are now so widely used, they have become a common cause of rhabdomyolysis, especially when used in high dose and in combination with ciclosporin.
- Aggressive fluid replacement and forced alkaline diuresis can prevent renal damage in rhabdomyolysis if started early enough.

CASE 29: COUGH AND JOINT PAINS

History

A 29-year-old man presents with a cough and some mild aches in the hands, wrists and ankles. The symptoms have been present for 2 months and have increased slightly over that time. Six weeks before, he had some soreness in his eyes, which resolved in 1 week.

The cough has been non-productive. He has noticed some skin lesions on the edge of his hairline and around his nostrils. Previously, he had been well, apart from an appendicectomy at the age of 17 years.

He was born in Trinidad and came to the United Kingdom at the age of 4 years. His two brothers and parents are well. He does not smoke, is a 'teetotaller' (a person who never drinks alcohol) and takes no recreational drugs. He works as a delivery driver and was regularly exercising until the past few weeks.

Examination

There is no deformity of the joints and no evidence of any acute inflammation. Examination of the respiratory and cardiovascular systems shows no abnormal findings. In the skin, there are some slightly raised areas on the edge of the hairline posteriorly and at the ala nasa. They are a little lighter than the rest of the skin.

🔍 INVESTIGATIONS

		Normal
Haemoglobin	13.5 g/dL	13.0–17.0 g/dL
Mean corpuscular volume (MCV)	88 fL	80–99 fL
White cell count	8.5×10^9/L	$3.5–11.0 \times 10^9$/L
Platelets	264×10^9/L	$150–440 \times 10^9$/L
Erythrocyte sedimentation rate (ESR)	34 mm	<10 mm/h
Sodium	140 mmol/L	135–145 mmol/L
Potassium	4.0 mmol/L	3.5–5.0 mmol/L
Urea	3.6 mmol/L	2.5–6.7 mmol/L
Creatinine	74 µmol/L	70–120 µmol/L
Bilirubin	14 mmol/L	3–17 mmol/L
Alkaline phosphatase	84 IU/L	30–300 IU/L
Alanine aminotransferase	44 IU/L	5–35 IU/L
Calcium	2.69 mmol/L	2.12–2.65 mmol/L
Phosphate	1.20 mmol/L	0.8–1.45 mmol/L

The chest radiograph is shown in Figure 29.1.

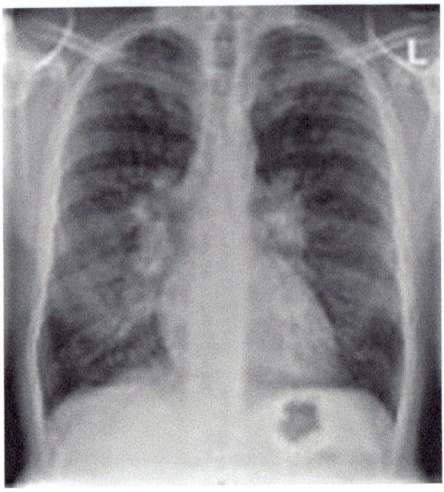

Figure 29.1 Chest radiograph.

? | QUESTIONS

- What is the likely diagnosis?
- How might this be confirmed?
- What is the management for this patient?

ANSWER 29

The likely diagnosis is sarcoidosis. The age is typical and sarcoidosis is more common in those of African-Caribbean origin. The chest radiograph shows bilateral hilar lymphadenopathy. The blood results show a slightly raised calcium level, which is related to vitamin D sensitivity in sarcoidosis, in which the granulomas hydroxylate 25-hydroxycholecalciferol to 1,25-dihydroxy-cholecalciferol. The ESR is raised and some of the liver enzymes are around the upper limit of normal. The skin lesions at the hairline and the nostrils (lupus pernio) are typical sites of cutaneous manifestations in sarcoidosis. The eye trouble 6 weeks earlier might also have been a manifestation of sarcoidosis, which can cause both anterior and posterior uveitis.

An alternative diagnosis that might explain the findings is tuberculosis. Tuberculosis can also cause hypercalcaemia, although this is much less common than in sarcoidosis. Tumours, especially lymphoma, might give this radiograph appearance but would not explain the other findings. The arthralgia (pains with no evidence of acute inflammation or deformity on examination) can occur in sarcoidosis or tuberculosis, but again is more common in sarcoidosis. The ESR is non-specific. Arthralgia without deformity in an African-Caribbean man raises the possibility of systemic lupus erythematosus (SLE), but this is much more common in women and would not cause bilateral hilar lymphadenopathy.

He is likely to have had the BCG (bacille Calmette–Guérin) vaccination at school, giving a degree of protection against tuberculosis. A tuberculin test should be positive after BCG, strongly positive in most cases of tuberculosis and negative in 80% of cases of sarcoidosis. The serum level of angiotensin-converting enzyme would be raised in over 80% of cases of sarcoidosis but often in tuberculosis also; the granuloma cells secrete this enzyme. A computed tomography (CT) scan of the chest will confirm the extent of the lymphadenopathy and show whether there is any involvement of the lung parenchyma. Biopsy of affected tissue (skin or another lesion) would confirm the clinical diagnosis, and findings such as the presence of Schaumann bodies, asteroid bodies and non-caseating granulomas would support the diagnosis. A bronchial or transbronchial lung biopsy at fibre-optic bronchoscopy would be another means of obtaining diagnostic histology. In patients with a cough and sarcoidosis, the bronchial mucosa itself often looks abnormal, and biopsy will provide the diagnosis. Lung function tests, which may show a restrictive ventilatory defect in sarcoidosis, and an electrocardiogram (ECG) should be performed as a baseline if the diagnosis is confirmed.

Oral or IV corticosteroids are indicated in acute flares of sarcoidosis. Steroid treatment would not be necessary for the hilar lymphadenopathy alone but would be indicated for the hypercalcaemia and possibly for the systemic symptoms. Topical corticosteroids are usually sufficient for treatment of skin lesions and ocular manifestations. Methotrexate, azathioprine, leflunomide or hydroxychloroquine can be used as corticosteroid-sparing agents in patients who do not tolerate high doses of corticosteroids, or as additional treatment in cases of unsatisfactory response to corticosteroids.

 KEY POINTS

- Sarcoidosis is more common in those of African-Caribbean heritage.
- Typical sites for skin lesions are around the nose and the hairline.
- Sarcoidosis is a systemic disease and can affect most parts of the body.

CASE 30: URINARY FREQUENCY

History

A 37-year-old man presents to his general practitioner (GP) with a 5-day history of urinary frequency, dysuria and urethral discharge. In the previous 24 hours, he has felt feverish and developed a painful right knee. He works in an international bank and frequently travels to East Asia and Australia, last returning from there 2 weeks ago. There is no relevant past medical or family history, and he takes no medication.

Examination

He looks unwell and has a temperature of 38.1°C. His heart rate is 90/min; blood pressure is 124/82 mmHg. Otherwise, examination of the cardiovascular, respiratory, abdominal and nervous systems is normal. His right knee is warm, swollen and tender. A moderate effusion is palpated with limitation of active and passive flexion. There is no skin rash and no oral mucosal abnormality. He has a cream-coloured urethral discharge.

🔍 INVESTIGATIONS

		Normal
Haemoglobin	17.1 g/dL	13.3–17.7 g/dL
White cell count	16.9 × 10⁹/L	3.9–10.6 × 10⁹/L
Platelets	222 × 10⁹/L	150–440 × 10⁹/L

Blood film: neutrophil leucocytosis
Urethral gram stain: multiple gram-negative diplococci seen.
CRP 186

His knee radiograph is shown in Figure 30.1.

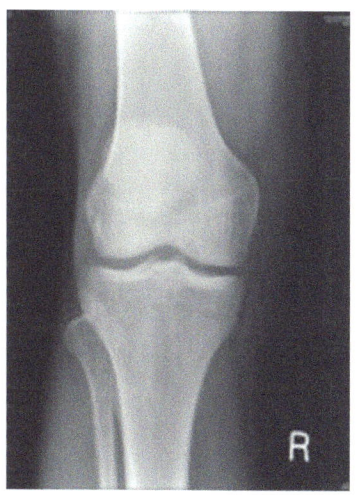

Figure 30.1 Radiograph of the right knee.

❓ QUESTIONS

- How would you investigate this patient?
- What is the likely diagnosis?
- How would you manage this patient?

DOI: 10.1201/9781003350934-33

ANSWER 30

The patient has acute gonorrhoea and gonococcal arthritis. The radiograph of the knee is normal. The diagnosis is made by microscopy which shows gram-negative diplococci. This must be sent for culture to identify the causative agent, *Neisseria gonorrhoeae*, and to attain sensitivities for definitive antibiotic treatment. Blood cultures must also be collected.

Immediate empirical treatment should be commenced, given the clinical picture, with ceftriaxone IV. Other agents such as ciprofloxacin may be used as an oral step-down once sensitivities are known, however, IV treatment is preferred in this case as there is joint involvement and the patient is unwell.

Septic monoarthritis is a complication of gonorrhoea. Patients should have joint aspiration or drainage to remove infected pus (this can also be sent for culture). Orthopaedic teams should be involved. Other metastatic complications are skin lesions and, rarely, perihepatitis, bacterial endocarditis and meningitis.

The patient disclosed that he had had unprotected sexual intercourse in Thailand and Singapore. He should therefore have a full sexual health screen including a human immunodeficiency virus (HIV) test and onward referral to the sexual health team.

 KEY POINTS

- All students and doctors should be confident in eliciting a sexual history.
- Accurate sexual histories are more likely when the patient feels confidence and empathy from the interviewer.
- Contact tracing is an important element of management of sexually transmitted disease.
- Consider extragenital symptoms of sexually transmitted infections. An important element of management is empirical treatment after cultures have been collected.

CASE 31: BACK PAIN

History

A 48-year-old woman presented to her general practitioner (GP) with a 3-month history of back pain in the mid-thoracic region. The pain is intermittent, worse at night and relieved by ibuprofen, which she bought herself. She has no other symptoms and no relevant past or family history. She has never smoked and drinks 10–12 units of alcohol most weeks. She works part-time stacking the shelves in a supermarket and is very active, being a competitive tennis and badminton player.

Examination

She looks well. She indicates that the pain is over the vertebrae at T5/6 but there is no tenderness, swelling or deformity. Her spinal movements are normal.

Her blood pressure is 136/76 mmHg. Cardiovascular, respiratory and abdomen examinations are normal.

 INVESTIGATIONS

Spinal radiograph was arranged and showed no abnormality. The full blood count, urea creatinine and electrolytes, calcium, alkaline phosphatase and phosphate were all normal, as was urine testing.

She was advised that the pain was musculoskeletal due to exertion at work and sport and she was prescribed diclofenac for the pain. She was advised to rest from her tennis and badminton.

After a few weeks of improvement, the pain began to get worse, becoming more severe, occurring for longer periods and seriously disturbing her sleep. She returned to her GP and examination was as before except that there was now some tenderness over her mid-thoracic spine. The GP arranged another radiograph of the spine (Figure 31.1).

Figure 31.1 Lateral radiograph of the thoracic spine.

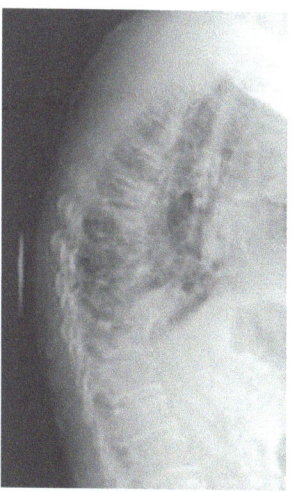

? **QUESTIONS**

- What is the abnormality in the radiograph?
- What are the likeliest causes?
- What further examination and investigations need to be done?

DOI: 10.1201/9781003350934-34

ANSWER 31

The radiograph shows collapse of the T6 vertebra. If there is nothing to suggest osteoporosis or trauma, then the commonest cause of this is a tumour metastasis. Tumours that most frequently metastasise to bone are carcinoma of the lung, prostate, thyroid, kidney and breast. Examination of the patient's breasts, not done before the radiograph result, revealed a firm mass, 1–1.5 cm diameter, in the tail of the left breast. Urgent biopsy confirmed a carcinoma, and she was referred to an oncologist for further management.

The common lesions affecting the lumbosacral and cervical spine (e.g., inflammation of ligaments and other soft tissues and lesions of the intervertebral discs) are much less common in the thoracic spine, and bony metastases should be considered as a cause of persistent pain in the thoracic spine in patients older than 50.

Review of the first radiograph, after the lesion was seen on the second film, still failed to identify a lesion, emphasising the need to repeat an investigation if there is sufficient clinical suspicion of an abnormality, even if an earlier investigation is normal.

Examination of the breasts in women should be part of routine examination, particularly after the age of 40 years, when the risk of breast cancer is significantly increased.

 KEY POINTS

- Pain in the thoracic vertebrae should raise the possibility of bony metastases in patients over the age of 40 years.
- Repeating previously normal or negative investigations is an important part of a patient's management when clinical diagnoses remain unconfirmed.

CASE 32: ACHES AND PAINS

History

A 72-year-old woman has felt non-specifically unwell for about 10 weeks. She feels stiff, especially when she gets up in the morning. She struggles to get out of bed by herself. She has difficulty lifting her hand to comb her hair and has needed help with some of her housework. She has also noticed some pain in her knees and fingers. She has lost 4 kg in weight and has noticed some sweats, which seem to occur at night. She has come to see her general practitioner (GP) because she has now developed a headache. This is a severe pain that has been persistent over the last 4–5 days. On direct questioning, she says that she has had some pain in her jaw when chewing. She has previously been fit with no significant past medical history. She lives alone. She has not smoked for 40 years, and she only drinks alcohol at Christmas. She takes no regular medication. She has tried some paracetamol, but this has not helped the headache.

Examination

She is thin. She is tender to palpation over parts of her scalp. Her blood pressure is 138/64 mmHg. Examination of her cardiovascular, respiratory and abdominal systems is normal. Power is slightly reduced in the proximal muscles of her arms and legs (MRC scale 4+: active movement against gravity and strong resistance). Neurological examination is otherwise normal.

🔍 INVESTIGATIONS

		Normal
Haemoglobin	10.3 g/dL	11.7–15.7 g/dL
Mean corpuscular volume (MCV)	87 fL	80–99 fL
White cell count	12.2 × 10⁹/L	3.5–11.0 × 10⁹/L
Platelets	377 × 10⁹/L	150–440 × 10⁹/L
Erythrocyte sedimentation rate (ESR)	91 mm/h	<10 mm/h
Sodium	139 mmol/L	135–145 mmol/L
Potassium	4.6 mmol/L	3.5–5.0 mmol/L
Urea	3.8 mmol/l	2.5–6./ mmol/L
Creatinine	102 µmol/L	70–120 µmol/L
Glucose	6.8 mmol/L	4.0–6.0 mmol/L
Albumin	38 g/L	35–50 g/L
Bilirubin	16 mmol/L	3–17 mmol/L
Alanine transaminase	85 IU/L	5–35 IU/L
Alkaline phosphatase	465 IU/L	30–300 IU/L
Creatine kinase	139 IU/L	25–195 IU/L

? QUESTIONS

- What is the diagnosis?
- What investigations would you consider for this patient?
- How would you manage this patient?

DOI: 10.1201/9781003350934-35

ANSWER 32

This woman has the typical clinical symptoms of polymyalgia rheumatica/giant cell arteritis. Most patients are over 65 years. The onset of symptoms is often sudden. Patients may present primarily with polymyalgia-type symptoms (proximal muscle pain and stiffness most marked in the mornings) or temporal arteritis symptoms (severe headaches with tenderness over the arteries involved). Patients may have systemic symptoms, such as general malaise, weight loss and night sweats. Characteristically, the ESR is very elevated (at least 40 mm/h), and there is a mild anaemia and leucocytosis. The liver enzymes are often slightly raised. In polymyalgia, the main symptoms are muscle stiffness and pain, which may simulate muscle weakness. The creatine kinase is normal, unlike in polymyositis.

The diagnosis of polymyalgia rheumatica is essentially a clinical one. A very elevated ESR is often seen and about 25% of patients with giant cell arteritis have polymyalgia. When there are headaches and giant cell arteritis is suspected, a temporal artery biopsy should be performed. However, the histology may be normal because the vessel involvement with inflammation is patchy. Nevertheless, a positive result provides reassurance about the diagnosis and the need for long-term steroids.

This patient has clear evidence of giant cell arteritis (also known as temporal arteritis, although other vessels are involved) and is at risk of irreversible visual loss due to either ischaemic damage to the ciliary arteries causing optic neuritis or central retinal artery occlusion. The patient should immediately be started on high-dose prednisolone based on the clinical picture before the biopsy is done. The results will not be affected by a few days of treatment and preservation of sight is the most important factor. The steroid dose should be slowly tapered according to clinical features and ESR but is likely to need to be continued for about 2 years. Bone protection measures should be part of the management.

! **DIFFERENTIAL DIAGNOSES OF PROXIMAL MUSCLE WEAKNESS AND STIFFNESS**

- Polymyositis
- Systemic vasculitis
- Systemic lupus erythematosus
- Parkinsonism
- Hypothyroidism/hyperthyroidism
- Osteomalacia

  KEY POINTS

- Polymyalgia rheumatica and giant cell arteritis often coexist.
- Patients with these conditions have markedly elevated ESR levels.
- There is a risk of blindness in giant cell arteritis, and steroids should be started immediately.

Section 4
CARDIOLOGY

CASE 33: CARDIAC IMPLANTABLE ELECTRONIC DEVICES

History

A 76-year-old man visiting from overseas is brought in unresponsive following a head injury. Whilst a computed tomography (CT) scan of the head is awaited, the emergency team has been unable to discern any past medical history.

Examination

Other than a Glasgow Coma Scale (GCS) of 6/15 (E2, V1, M3), vital signs are within normal limits. Clinical examination reveals three scars: a midline sternotomy, a long, fine scar over the right radial artery and a 2-inch incision below the left clavicle with a hard, pre-pectoral mass underlying. On auscultation, heart sounds are normal and the lung fields are clear. Examination of the lower limbs is unremarkable.

 INVESTIGATIONS

A chest radiograph and electrocardiogram (ECG) have been performed (Figures 33.1 and 33.2).

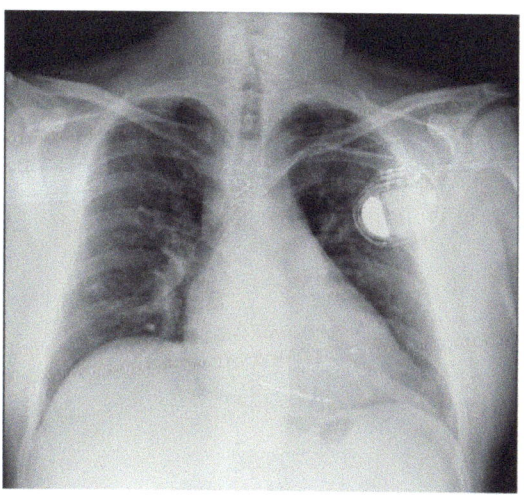

Figure 33.1 Chest radiograph.

DOI: 10.1201/9781003350934-37

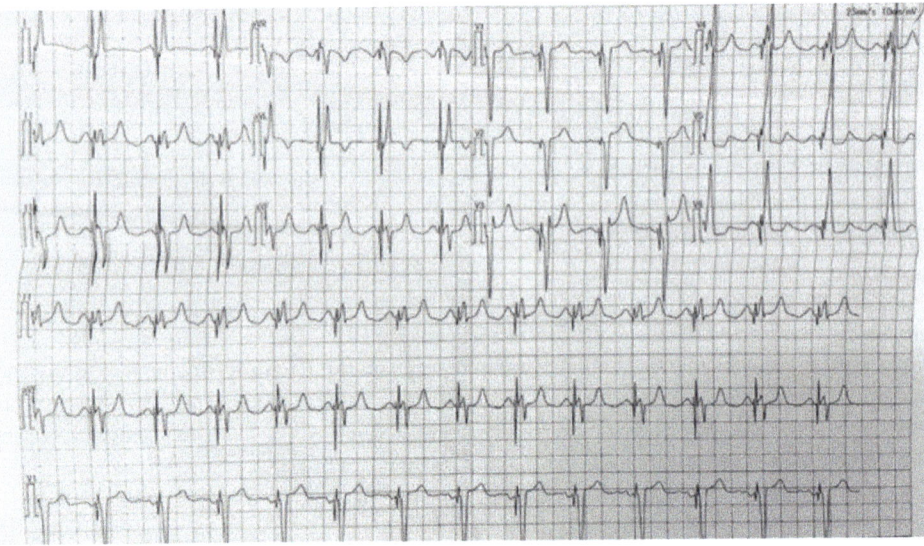

Figure 33.2 12-lead electrocardiogram.

? | **QUESTIONS**

- What is the most likely underlying cardiac history?
- What device does the chest radiograph show?
- What does the ECG show?

ANSWER 33

In the absence of a clinical history, the differential diagnosis for a mid-line sternotomy scar is broad and includes valvular or aortic interventions, coronary artery bypass grafting (CABG), repaired congenital heart disease and other non-cardiac mediastinal procedures (such as thymectomy). On examination, clues as to the underlying diagnosis may be evident on inspection of the peripheries (such as saphenous vein or radial artery bypass graft scars) or on auscultation (such as the click of a metallic valve replacement). Note that the absence of vein grafting scars on the lower limbs does not preclude CABG; the radial arteries and both internal mammary arteries can be mobilised to achieve multivessel revascularisation if required. Likewise, surgical graft clips are not always well-visualised on a chest radiograph.

An implanted cardiac device is clearly seen on the chest radiograph. Identifying the nature of the device by the generator alone can be challenging and, although algorithms do exist to assist with this, it is the leads that tend to provide the most useful information. A lead is clearly seen in both the right atrium and right ventricle (RV). This device is therefore at least a dual-chamber pacemaker. However, the device generator itself is large, and the right ventricular lead has a thickened segment near its insertion in the RV apex; this is the shock coil of a defibrillator. The device is therefore some sort of implantable cardioverter-defibrillator (ICD), and the (subtle) presence of a smaller third lead projected over the left ventricle (positioned in a branch vein of the coronary sinus) clarifies that this device is also capable of cardiac resynchronisation therapy (CRT). This device is therefore a CRT-D; a complex device with leads sensing and pacing the right atrium and both ventricles, with defibrillator capability. Accordingly, whilst simple pacemakers will result in a broad left bundle branch block (LBBB) during paced rhythm, CRT devices are designed to coordinate cardiac depolarisation in a manner that improves interventricular synchrony and therefore contractility. As such, the ECG here shows a relatively narrow QRS, a hallmark of biventricular pacing.

To have had any kind of defibrillator implanted, at this age, it is reasonable to assume that this patient has severe left ventricular impairment and the presence of CRT functionality suggests concomitant heart failure symptoms with a broad underlying QRS complex. In light of the previous sternotomy and radial graft scars, it seems most likely that the patient has a history of ischaemic heart disease requiring a CABG, with subsequent severe systolic dysfunction; this is a common indication for CRT-D insertion.

 KEY POINTS

- In patients unable to provide a clinical history, or without a pacemaker identification card, an ECG and a chest radiograph can be used to distinguish different types of cardiac devices.
- A paced QRS that is narrow, or non-LBBB, is suggestive of a CRT device.
- Saphenous vein graft scars are not always present in CABG patients.

History

A 23-year-old nurse comes to see you in clinic with recurrent palpitations. She describes monthly episodes of her heart suddenly racing for a few minutes. The symptoms are associated with profound anxiety and can provoke light-headedness, but they resolve spontaneously. She has never been syncopal and has no family history of sudden cardiac death. She is asthmatic requiring as-needed salbutamol only. She reports that she drinks at least 4 cups of coffee daily and is a non-smoker.

Examination

On examination, she is well-perfused with a regular radial pulse of 75/min. Oxygen saturations are 99% on air. Her jugular venous pressure is not elevated and there are no murmurs on auscultation.

🔍 **INVESTIGATIONS**

Her electrocardiogram (ECG) is shown in Figure 34.1.

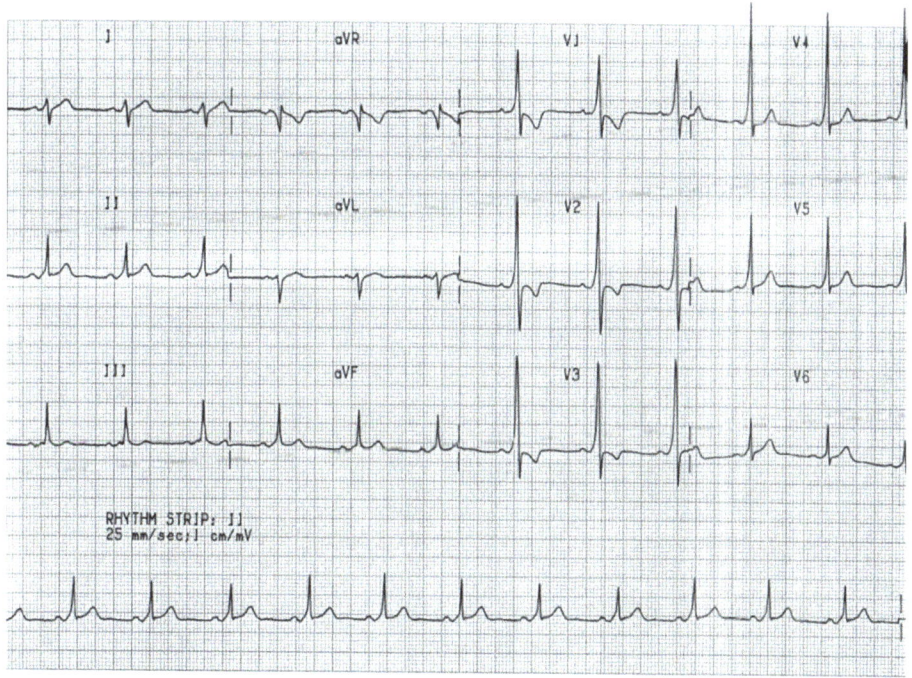

Figure 34.1 12-lead electrocardiogram.

❓ **QUESTIONS**

- What does the ECG show?
- Why can this condition be dangerous?
- What is the definitive management in symptomatic patients?

ANSWER 34

The ECG demonstrates a short PR interval merging into each QRS complex with a slurred upstroke (a 'delta wave'), which is best appreciated in leads V2–3. This suggests pre-excitation which, when combined with a history of palpitations, is pathognomonic of Wolff-Parkinson-White (WPW) syndrome. This ECG appearance is the result of an additional electrical ('accessory') pathway in the heart, which bypasses the AV node, forming a circuit that can sustain episodes of atrio-ventricular re-entry tachycardia (AVRT), the likely cause of this patient's symptoms. The Arruda algorithm, which examines delta wave morphology, suggests that this particular accessory pathway is in the left lateral position.

During tachycardia, accessory pathways support AVRT either by conducting from the ventricles back to the atria ('orthodromic AVRT') or, less commonly, from the atria down to the ventricles ('antidromic AVRT'). Importantly, the conduction characteristics of accessory pathways differ broadly between patients. In the above case, the finding of pre-excitation verifies that the pathway can conduct from the atria down to the ventricles during sinus rhythm (known as 'antero-grade conduction'), confirming that this is a 'manifest' accessory pathway. As such, the concern is that, in the event of an atrial arrhythmia (such as atrial fibrillation [AF]), the atrial impulses could be conducted anterogradely past the atrioventricular (AV) node and into the ventricle, causing an extremely rapid pre-excited arrhythmia (i.e., antidromic AVRT). By contrast, other accessory pathways only conduct from the ventricles back to the atria (known as 'retrograde conduction' through a 'concealed' pathway). These concealed pathways can still sustain the less dangerous orthodromic AVRT, but they do not cause pre-excitation on an ECG. Finally, certain manifest pathways are only capable of conducting up to a certain heart rate; in such cases, loss of pre-excitation can be seen during a treadmill test, for example. This is diagnostic of a 'safe' accessory pathway, which would be incapable of rapid conduction during an atrial arrhythmia.

With this in mind, in symptomatic individuals, the definitive management is to offer an invasive electrophysiology study to assess the direction and speed of pathway conduction. If the pathway is found to be capable of rapid conduction (i.e., is an 'unsafe' pathway), ablation can then be performed at the same sitting.

 KEY POINTS

- The combination of a delta wave and palpitations suggests WPW syndrome.
- Accessory pathways have variable conduction properties; some can cause life-threatening arrhythmias.
- Ablation is the definitive management in symptomatic patients, and is also mandated in pre-excited patients with high-risk occupations (such as military pilots).

History

A 24-year-old man is admitted under the medical team with pyelonephritis. He has no significant past medical history, but reports he recently attended his young cousin's funeral, who died suddenly in his sleep. He is an endurance runner with an excellent exercise tolerance.

Examination

On examination, the patient looks clammy and flushed. There is tenderness at the left renal angle. Cardiovascular examination is otherwise normal. His temperature is 38.4°C, pulse 101/min, blood pressure 104/72 mmHg, respiratory rate 20/min and oxygen saturations are 98% on air.

 INVESTIGATIONS

His urine dip is significant for +++ leukocytes and ++ nitrites. An electrocardiogram (ECG) is shown in Figure 35.1.

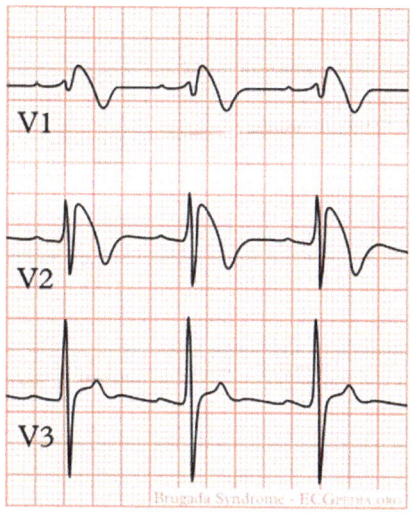

Figure 35.1 Electrocardiogram whilst febrile.

A repeat ECG on the ward, once the patient is afebrile, is shown in Figure 35.2.

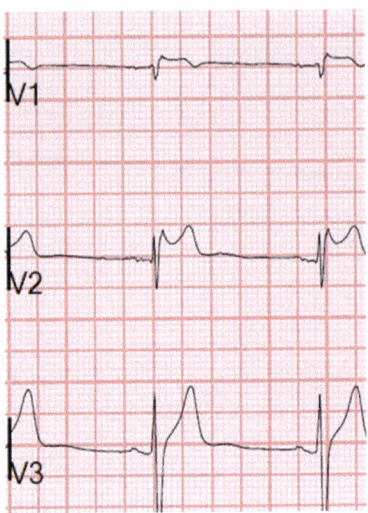

Figure 35.2 Electrocardiogram whilst afebrile.

? | **QUESTIONS**

- What do the ECGs show?
- Why have the ECGs changed?
- How should he be managed from a cardiovascular perspective?

ANSWER 35

The first trace shows the coved ST elevation typical of a type 1 Brugada ECG pattern. Brugada syndrome is a sodium channelopathy associated with life-threatening ventricular arrhythmias. The diagnosis is made based on the presence of a type 1 ECG pattern and clinical characteristics, which include documented ventricular arrhythmias, syncope or a family history of premature sudden cardiac death. Type 2 and 3 Brugada ECG patterns are not diagnostic of the syndrome in isolation but can be provoked into a type 1 pattern by medication (such as sodium channel blockers) or – as in this case – during fever, when higher temperatures accentuate the loss of function of the sodium channel current.

For all patients with Brugada pattern ECGs, advice should be given around the avoidance of certain medications and the prompt treatment of any fevers with anti-pyretic medication. Further management is guided by Inherited Arrhythmia specialists, who will complete risk stratification with the use of Holter monitors, genetic testing (with mutations in the *SCN5A* gene having the strongest association) and, in cases of diagnostic uncertainty, Ajmaline testing, in which a sodium channel blocker is injected to try and provoke a classical type 1 ECG. Given this patient's ECG findings and suspicious family history, all of his first-degree relatives should be screened for the condition. For high-risk patients with a definitive diagnosis of Brugada syndrome, such as those with a resting type 1 Brugada ECG pattern and a documented ventricular arrhythmia, an implantable cardioverter defibrillator (ICD) is recommended to protect against sudden cardiac death.

Contemporary ICDs may be transvenous (in which at least one lead is inserted inside the heart) or subcutaneous (S-ICD), in which a single lead is positioned under the skin on top of the sternum. By virtue of having a lead inside the heart, transvenous ICDs have additional functionality in that they may also function as pacemakers. However, lead-related complications (such as endocarditis) can be grave and, therefore, in patients who would not benefit from pacing capability, an S-ICD may be preferable. In those Brugada syndrome patients with repeated ventricular arrhythmias, medical therapy with Quinidine or an ablation procedure can also be offered.

 KEY POINTS

- Coved ST elevation is the key feature of a type 1 Brugada ECG pattern; these changes can be provoked by fevers and by certain medications (such as sodium channel blockers).
- All patients should be educated regarding fever management and the importance of avoiding drugs which may exacerbate the condition.
- Screening and risk stratification is available in specialist cardiac centres.

CASE 36: CHEST PAIN

History

A 39-year-old fireman develops crushing chest pain shortly after attending a house fire. He is previously fit and well, but he has a strong family history of premature coronary artery disease, with his father suffering a myocardial infarction at age 51.

Examination

Upon arrival to the emergency department, he looks unwell; capillary refill time is 3 seconds peripherally and the jugular venous pulse is raised at 6 cm above the sternal notch. There are no murmurs on auscultation, however there are bibasal crepitations. Heart rate is 110/min and blood pressure 98/53 mmHg. He is afebrile but he is tachypnoeic with oxygen saturations of 93% on air.

 INVESTIGATIONS

His electrocardiogram (ECG) shows anterior ST elevation and his point-of-care troponin blood test is 4000 ng/l. Bedside echocardiogram shows complete akinesis of all the mid- and apical segments of the left ventricle, with overall severely impaired systolic function. He is therefore given aspirin 300 mg and ticagrelor 180 mg, and undergoes emergency angiography via the right radial artery; this shows smooth, unobstructed coronary arteries and, hence, no intervention is performed. Recovering in the Coronary Care Unit 3 days later, a repeat bedside echocardiogram is entirely normal.

? **QUESTIONS**

- What is the diagnosis?
- Was the patient's initial management appropriate?
- What is the prognosis?

ANSWER 36

Takotsubo cardiomyopathy is named after the Japanese Octopus pot which the afflicted left ventricle resembles on echocardiography (or invasive ventriculography, shown in Figure 36.1). The condition is known by a variety of other names including stress cardiomyopathy, apical ballooning syndrome or broken-heart syndrome, and typically occurs in situations of high stress whereby a pooling of cardiac catecholamines stuns and frequently dilates the distal left ventricle. The combination of chest pain, raised troponin and ischaemic ECG findings (often ST elevation) can mimic an ST-elevation myocardial infarction (STEMI) and, as in this case, it is entirely appropriate to manage patients as per a STEMI pathway in the first instance (i.e., with antiplatelets and emergent angiography). Takotsubo cardiomyopathy often resolves entirely, usually within 6 weeks; angiotensin-converting enzyme (ACE) inhibitors and beta-blockers may assist with cardiac remodelling, although there is no evidence of mortality benefit from the latter.

This patient had clinical features of acute left ventricular decompensation on arrival. In the context of chest pain, acute coronary syndrome is the most common cause of acute heart failure, however inflammatory cardiomyopathies (such as myocarditis) or aortic syndromes (such as aortic dissection) should also be considered. In severe cases, patients with Takotsubo cardiomyopathy may present in cardiogenic shock. In such instances, inotropic support may be required, however catecholamine administration (such as adrenaline) should be avoided.

Having historically been considered a benign condition, recent data suggest outcomes in Takotsubo cardiomyopathy are comparable to those in acute coronary syndrome, with in-hospital mortality ranging from 2% to 8%. Those with physical triggers (such as a recent operation or illness) rather than emotional triggers have the least favourable prognosis, and recurrence of the condition is seen in about 5% of patients.

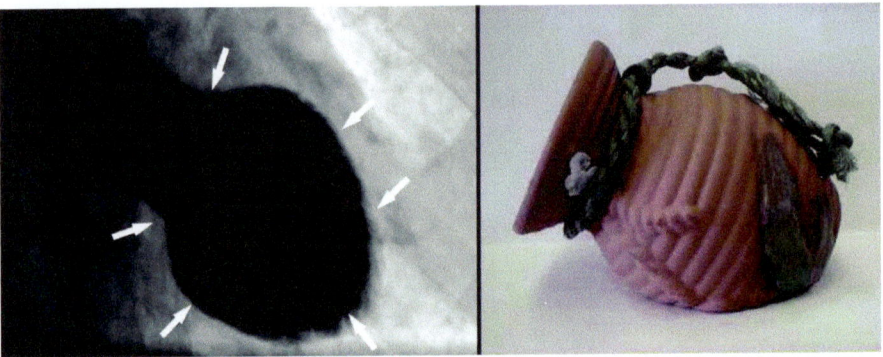

Figure 36.1 Left: invasive ventriculogram. **Right:** a Takotsubo (Japanese Octopus pot).

🔑 **KEY POINTS**

- An acute cardiomyopathy can follow episodes of extreme physical or emotional stress, however, an acute coronary syndrome should be excluded first, and empirical treatment (and investigation) for an ischaemic event is often the safest way to proceed.
- The systolic dysfunction associated with Takotsubo cardiomyopathy can be profound but is usually transient.
- Adrenaline administration should be avoided (and indeed can be causative) in cases of Takotsubo cardiomyopathy.

History

A 19-year-old woman collapses at a firework display. She recovers spontaneously and is taken to the emergency department. She says she has no definite past medical history but does recall previous dizzy spells. These are occasionally very severe when she first wakes up in the morning. She takes the combined oral contraceptive pill, but no other regular medications. She was adopted as a baby and is not able to provide a detailed family history. She drinks 20 units of alcohol per week and is a non-smoker.

Examination

Cardiovascular and neurological examinations are normal.

 INVESTIGATIONS

A bedside echocardiogram in emergency department shows a structurally normal heart.
Her electrocardiogram (ECG) is shown in Figure 37.1.
Her electrolyte panel is normal.

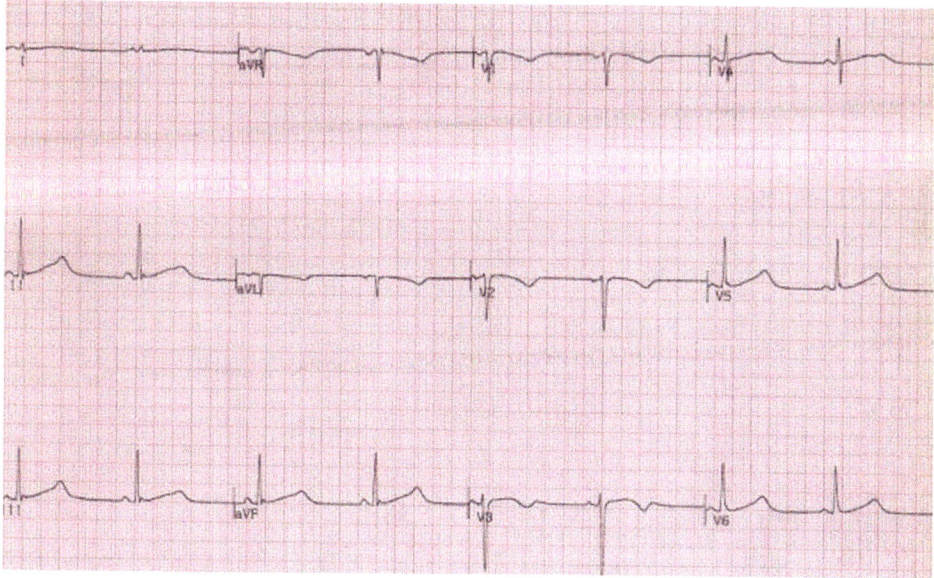

Figure 37.1 12-lead electrocardiogram.

? **QUESTIONS**

- What is the most likely diagnosis?
- What tests can be used for risk stratification?
- What are the long-term treatment options?

ANSWER 37

This ECG shows a markedly prolonged QT interval. The patient does not take any QT-prolonging medications and has a normal electrolyte panel, therefore, her presentation is likely to constitute congenital (as opposed to acquired) long QT syndrome (LQTS). The finding of a 'double-peaked' T wave (seen most clearly in lead V4), is suggestive of type 2 LQTS, however, note that this ECG morphology is also seen in acquired (e.g., drug-induced) long QT, which affects the same *hERG*-encoded potassium channel. In the context of this ECG, the history of dizziness and syncope provoked by loud noises (e.g., fireworks, alarm clocks) is suspicious for episodes of non-sustained ventricular arrhythmia, particularly polymorphic ventricular tachycardia (VT). These particular triggers are again classical for type 2 LQTS, but can be associated with any long QT phenotype.

There are more than a dozen types of LQTS; type 1 is the most common, with an ECG characterised by broad-based T waves, followed by type 2, and then the rarer type 3, in which T waves are characteristically very late and sharply peaked.

An acquired long QT interval is most commonly associated with certain medications, including the typical anti-psychotics (such as chlorpromazine), quinolone and macrolide antibiotics (such as moxifloxacin or erythromycin) and anti-arrhythmic drugs (such as sotalol, amiodarone or quinidine).

In cases of diagnostic uncertainty, exercise testing can be performed to look for appropriate QT shortening, and genetic testing is now available (with *KCNQ1*, *KCNH2* and *SCN5A* mutations most commonly implicated). Holter monitoring may be used to examine the presence and morphology of any ventricular ectopics. Those which very closely follow the preceding QRS are known as 'short-coupled' ectopics, which confer a particularly high risk of precipitating an 'R on T' event, hence polymorphic VT.

With regard to treatment, in those patients presenting with electrical storms, the QT interval may be shortened acutely with positive chronotropic medications (such as isoprenaline), or with temporary pacing. In the long term, management involves conservative measures such as avoiding particular triggers (e.g., swimming), ensuring adequate electrolyte supplementation and medications such as beta-blockers (with nadolol having the strongest evidence of benefit). In high-risk patients, implantable cardioverter defibrillators (ICDs) are recommended.

 KEY POINTS

- Even when the syncopal patient presents in sinus rhythm, the diagnosis can still be arrhythmogenic syncope; be vigilant for channelopathies on a 12 lead ECG.
- A double-peaked T wave can be suggestive of either acquired long QT or type 2 LQTS.
- There are dozens of medications which prolong the QT interval, but it is worth remembering particular culprit classes, such as antipsychotics, antibiotics and antiarrhythmic drugs.

CASE 38: DIZZY SPELLS

History

A 52-year-old woman presents with sudden onset dizziness and palpitations. She has a history of type 2 diabetes mellitus on insulin therapy and is also on treatment for hypertension with amlodipine. She ordinarily reports a preserved exercise tolerance and she is free of chest pain. She is a non-smoker. After 2 hours, her symptoms have not resolved, therefore, she attends her local emergency department.

Examination

On examination, she looks grey and clammy. Her pulse is 172/min and her blood pressure is 78/40 mmHg. Oxygen saturations are 93% on air. On examination, she has a low-volume radial pulse with no evidence of peripheral oedema. There are no obvious murmurs, however there are bibasal crepitations.

🔍 INVESTIGATIONS

Figure 38.1 shows her electrocardiogram (ECG).

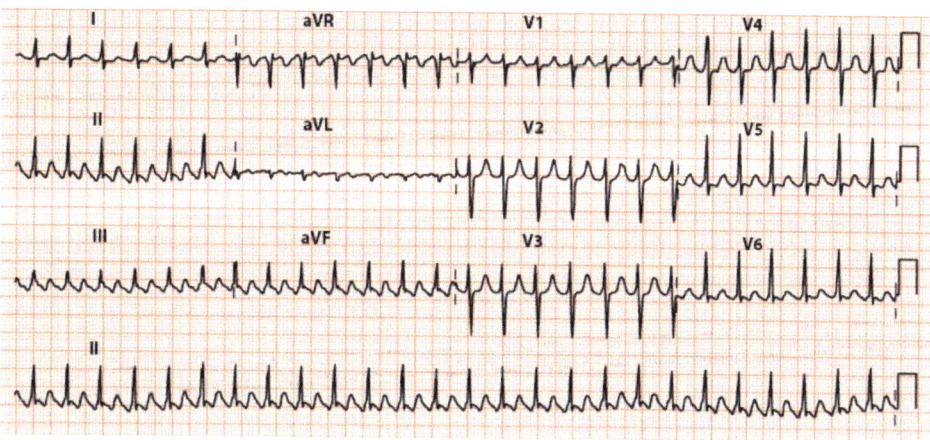

Figure 38.1 12-lead electrocardiogram.

? QUESTIONS

- What rhythm is shown?
- What treatment options are available acutely in stable patients?
- What interventional treatments are available in the long term?

DOI: 10.1201/9781003350934-42

ANSWER 38

This ECG shows a regular, narrow complex tachycardia which does not look like sinus rhythm. As such, this must be a form of supraventricular tachycardia (SVT). On closer inspection, there are two p waves seen before each QRS complex, in keeping with some form of atrial tachycardia. These p waves are positive in V1 and negative in the inferior leads and, therefore, this episode of SVT appears to be typical atrial flutter.

This patient has a tachyarrhythmia with evidence of haemodynamic instability, and therefore – as per the UK Resuscitation Council's Adult Life Support guidelines – the initial treatment is synchronised direct current (DC) cardioversion. In this scenario, a suitably trained practitioner should be contacted to assist with sedation, and a synchronised shock should be administered via an external defibrillator. Taking the time to enable the synchronisation (or 'sync') feature on the defibrillator is essential; this instructs the defibrillator to line up the delivery of energy with the R wave, which reduces the risk of accidentally shocking on the T wave and causing polymorphic ventricular tachycardia.

In the stable patient with an atrial arrhythmia of recent onset, an assessment must first be made regarding the risk of thromboembolism. In the absence of anticoagulation, sustained atrial arrhythmias can lead to thrombus formation in the left atrial appendage which carries a risk of embolic stroke; this risk is especially high in the period following cardioversion. As such, in those presenting with atrial arrhythmias and symptoms of >48 hours' duration, a period of at least 3 weeks' anticoagulation is recommended prior to any attempt at restoring sinus rhythm. However, in those for whom early cardioversion is still preferred, a transoesophageal echocardiogram can be performed to exclude thrombus in the left atrial appendage. As per the NICE guidelines, anticoagulation should be offered to all patients with a CHA_2DS_2VASc score of ≥ 2.

For those patients with low thromboembolic risk (i.e., symptoms <48 hours' duration, or at least 3 weeks' therapeutic anticoagulation), cardioversion can also be attempted chemically with anti-arrhythmic medication. Intravenous amiodarone is preferred (or, if available, ibutilide), whereas flecainide should be avoided due to the risk of slowing the atrial rate such that the atrioventricular (AV) node can conduct 1:1, accelerating the tachycardia. If achieving sinus rhythm is not safe or desirable, heart rate control with AV nodal blocking drugs, such as beta-blockers or non-dihydropyridine calcium channel blockers (e.g., verapamil), should be instituted aiming for a heart rate persistently <110/min. Digoxin may also be used for rate control in patients with features of left ventricular systolic dysfunction.

Typical atrial flutter occurs as a result of an electrical re-entry circuit around the cavo-tricuspid isthmus in the right atrium. Catheter ablation – in which a line of radiofrequency energy is delivered across this isthmus – is the definitive long-term treatment for patients in whom sinus rhythm is preferred and carries a long-term success rate of >90%.

🔑 **KEY POINTS**

- Regardless of aetiology, patients presenting with a tachyarrhythmia and associated adverse clinical features – such as hypotension or pulmonary oedema – warrant emergency electrical cardioversion.
- Always assess thromboembolic risk – and therefore the need for anticoagulation – in patients with atrial arrhythmias.
- Catheter ablation is the definitive long-term treatment for atrial flutter.

CASE 39: MURMUR

History

A general practitioner (GP) phones you about a 23-year-old woman who has recently moved to the UK. Whilst she is asymptomatic, at registration, she reports a past medical history of a 'heart problem', and she provides the results of diagnostic tests performed overseas.

Examination

The GP reports that the patient has a normal blood pressure and looks well. Radial pulse volume is normal, however, the jugular venous pressure is markedly raised. On auscultation, there is a loud, harsh pansystolic murmur across the precordium.

 INVESTIGATIONS

Her previous investigations include the results of a right heart catheterisation study (Table 39.1).

TABLE 39.1 **Summary of findings from a right heart catheterisation study**

Sampling site	Oxygen saturations
Inferior vena cava	74%
Right atrium	74%
Right ventricle	91%
Aortic root	94%

? **QUESTIONS**

- What is the most likely diagnosis?
- What variations of this condition exist?
- When might this condition need treatment?

ANSWER 39

A right heart catheterisation can provide useful information on cardiac output, pulmonary pressure and the presence of any significant shunts. In this case, there is a noticeable step up in oxygenation seen from the right atrium to the right ventricle. This suggests that oxygenated blood is being received from the left ventricle which, especially in the setting of a harsh, pansystolic murmur, suggests a ventricular septal defect (VSD) with left-to-right shunt. Blood flow across VSDs is typically very fast, with a significant pressure gradient and, as a result, the associated murmur is often loud, high-pitched, harsh in quality and audible across the precordium. A thrill may be palpable and features of right ventricular overload (such as raised jugular venous pressure) may be evident. Importantly, S2 is usually loud, distinguishing this murmur from that of severe aortic stenosis, which has ejection systolic timing and in which S2 is absent.

Several subtypes of VSD exist. Perimembranous VSDs, with the defect located near the membranous portion of the ventricular septum just below the aortic and tricuspid valves, are the most common. VSDs through the lower part of the septum are known as 'muscular'; these are usually small and are not always congenital – they may be acquired in late-presenting septal myocardial infarction, for example. Inlet (or atrioventricular [AV] canal) VSDs and outlet (or conal) VSDs are rarer, and both may be associated with other congenital abnormalities, such as the outlet VSD seen in Tetralogy of Fallot.

Over time, additional blood in the pulmonary circulation increases venous return to the left heart, which can result in left ventricular overload. Eventually, large, persistent left-to-right shunts may lead to irreversible changes in the pulmonary vascular endothelium and, consequently, pulmonary hypertension. Once the pressure in the pulmonary circulation surpasses that of the systemic circulation, shunt direction can change to right-to-left such that deoxygenated blood passes into the systemic circulation. The resulting hypoxemia results in the clinical finding of cyanosis; this is Eisenmenger syndrome.

VSD closure can be achieved by both surgical and transcatheter techniques. If there is evidence of left ventricular overload but pulmonary hypertension has not yet developed, closure is recommended regardless of symptoms. Closure should also be considered in those with associated aortic regurgitation, recurrent endocarditis or in left ventricular overload and non-severe pulmonary hypertension with a persistent left-to-right shunt. Upon the development of severe pulmonary hypertension or Eisenmenger physiology, VSD closure is no longer recommended.

 KEY POINTS

- Ventricular septal defects may not always cause symptoms, even in those patients with a loud murmur.
- A right heart catheterisation study can investigate the haemodynamic consequences of shunt and is the gold standard for the assessment of pulmonary hypertension.
- Left ventricular overload is an important prognostic feature and is a key consideration in decisions regarding VSD closure.

CASE 40: SHORTNESS OF BREATH

History

An 82-year-old man attends the emergency department describing a 2-week history of worsening shortness of breath and intermittent palpitations. He is now breathless on minimal exertion, and the palpitations – which last up to 30 seconds – are rapid, regular and associated with presyncope.

Five months ago, he suffered an ST elevation myocardial infarction (STEMI) requiring emergency percutaneous coronary intervention to his left anterior descending artery. He recalls that he had an ultrasound of his heart prior to discharge which showed 'severely reduced pumping function'. He currently takes aspirin 75 mg, clopidogrel 75 mg, atorvastatin 80 mg, ramipril 5 mg, bisoprolol 3.75 mg and eplerenone 25 mg.

Examination

On examination, his pulse is 70/min and blood pressure 108/66 mmHg. He is visibly tachypnoeic. Jugular venous pressure is markedly elevated and there is a sustained apical heave on palpation of the precordium. There is a soft pansystolic murmur which radiates apically.

 INVESTIGATIONS

Blood tests show a troponin of 14 ng/l and an NT-proBNP of 4,500 pg/ml. Chest radiograph is shown in Figure 40.1.

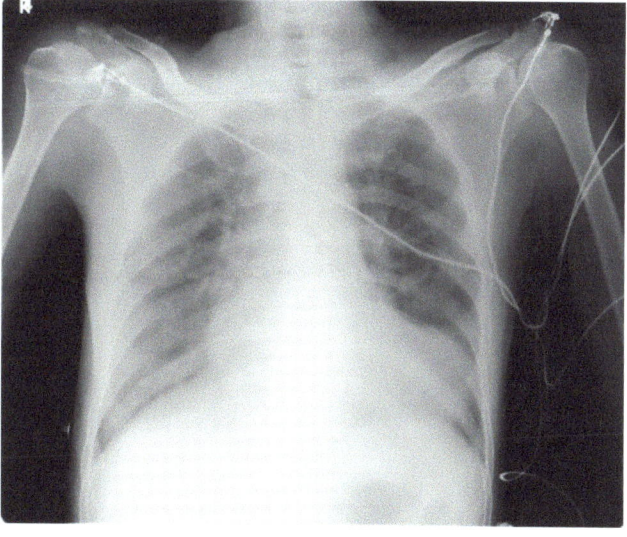

Figure 40.1 Chest radiograph.

? **QUESTIONS**

- What does the chest radiograph show?
- How might this finding be implicated in his palpitations?
- How could his long-term medical treatment be optimised?

DOI: 10.1201/9781003350934-44

ANSWER 40

The chest radiograph shows a 'boot-shaped heart' which, given the patient's recent myocardial infarction, most likely represents a left ventricular aneurysm. A damaged area of myocardium can form an internal pocket within the ventricle, within which blood (and frequently thrombi) collects. Whilst infarction is the most common cause, these aneurysms may also be congenital, cardiomyopathic or infective in aetiology. Echocardiogram is the most useful bedside test to confirm the diagnosis and, in the acutely unwell patient, can distinguish aneurysms from pseudo-aneurysms (or 'false' aneurysms, Figure 40.2), in which ruptured myocardium is contained within an outpouching of pericardium; the latter may require emergency surgery.

In addition to thrombi, complications associated with left ventricular aneurysms include ventricular arrhythmias, the likely cause of this patient's palpitations and presyncope. In particular, an aneurysm neck can provide part of the re-entry circuit required to sustain ventricular tachycardia (VT). In this patient's case, if VT is proven, medical management with beta-blockers and amiodarone would be preferred, with catheter ablation a second-line (and high-risk) strategy if the VT is poorly tolerated and refractory to anti-arrhythmic drugs.

The patient's clinical status and blood tests support the diagnosis of decompensated heart failure. As such, following acute stabilisation, his long-term medications should be reviewed. There is now compelling evidence for SGLT2 inhibitors (such as dapagliflozin) for heart failure patients both with and without a reduced ejection fraction. In addition, sacubitril-valsartan (Entresto) also improves outcomes in this population and, after a 36-hour washout period, could substitute this patient's angiotensin-converting enzyme (ACE) inhibitor. Importantly, for patients whose

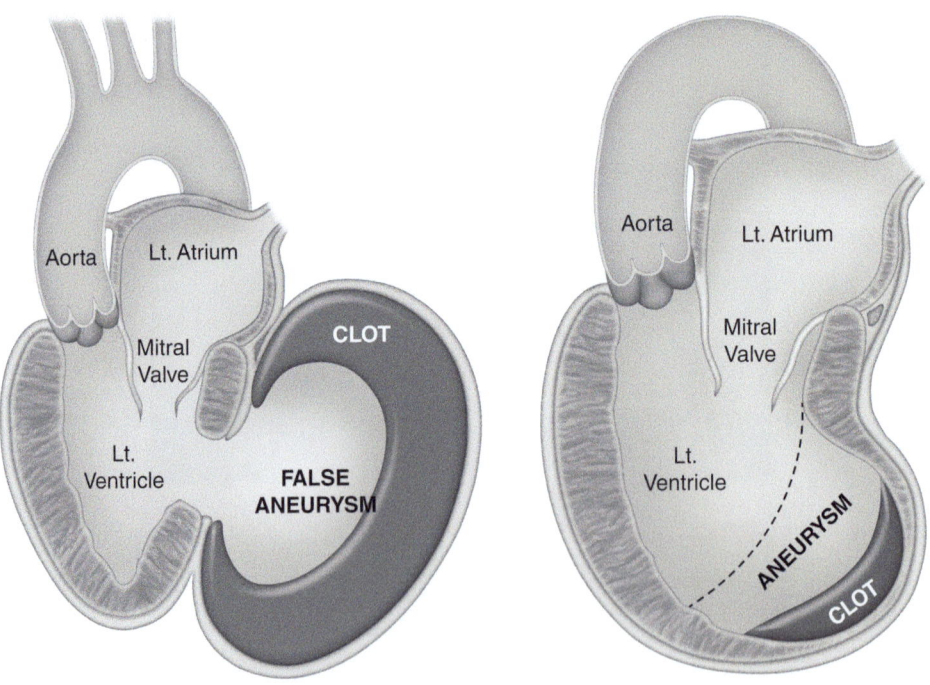

Figure 40.2 Distinction between ventricular pseudo-aneurysms (or 'false' aneurysms) (left) and aneurysms (right).

ejection fraction remains <35% despite optimal medical therapy, an implantable cardioverter-defibrillator (ICD) should be implanted as primary prevention against sudden cardiac death. If left bundle branch block (>130 ms) is also evident, a defibrillator with cardiac resynchronisation capability (i.e., a CRT-D) should be offered.

🔑 KEY POINTS

- A boot-shaped heart on chest radiograph should trigger investigation into the possibility of a left ventricular aneurysm, especially in patients with previous myocardial infarction.
- Echocardiography can help distinguish between aneurysms and pseudo-aneurysms, which are medical emergencies.
- Alongside beta-blockers and mineralocorticoid receptor antagonists, the more recently developed angiotensin-receptor neprilysin inhibitors (e.g., sacubitril-valsartan) and SGLT2 inhibitors (e.g., dapagliflozin) form part of the 'four pillars' of medical therapy for heart failure patients.

CASE 41: FATIGUE

History

A 45-year-old man presents with a 2-week history of progressive fatigue and night sweats which first developed a few days after a dental procedure. On arrival in the emergency department, he is noted to have a cough productive of pink sputum.

Examination

On examination, he feels warm and has a bounding, rapid radial pulse, with a blood pressure of 171/57 mmHg. His carotid arteries distend markedly before emptying rapidly. A soft murmur is heard after the second heart sound.

 INVESTIGATIONS

His C-reactive protein is 232 mg/l and white cell count is 18 ×10⁹/l. Chest radiograph shows evidence of pulmonary venous congestion.

? **QUESTIONS**

- What murmur is being described?
- What criteria are used to support the most likely diagnosis?
- When should surgical intervention be considered?

ANSWER 41

This patient's clinical history is suspicious for infective endocarditis, with examination demonstrating classical features of significant aortic regurgitation. Following systole, the aortic valve closes (this is a component of the second heart sound) and, in the case of an incompetent valve, blood regurgitates back into the ventricle with an associated murmur. This repeated additional blood volume leads to a large ventricular stroke volume (with high systolic blood pressure and exaggerated arterial pulsations) but with abrupt reversal of blood flow in early diastole. The resulting collapsing pulse can be appreciated as a number of eponymous clinical signs, including Corrigan's 'dancing' carotid pulsations, and gives rise to a wide pulse pressure.

The diagnosis of infective endocarditis is supported by the Duke criteria:

Pathological criteria (definitive diagnosis):

1. Identification of microorganisms in a vegetation.
2. Culprit lesions (vegetations or abscesses) confirmed on histological examination as active endocarditis.

Major criteria:

1. Positive blood cultures with a typical microorganism. For example, two separate cultures identifying *Staphylococcus aureus*, Viridans-group streptococcus or one of the HACEK group (*Haemophilus*, *Aggregatibacter*, *Cardiobacterium*, *Eikenella* and *Kingella*).
2. Evidence of endocardial involvement: Echocardiogram demonstrating a vegetation or new valvular regurgitation.

Minor criteria:

1. Predisposing cardiac condition (such as a congenital valvular lesion) or intravenous drug use.
2. Fever.
3. Vascular phenomena (such as septic emboli or conjunctival haemorrhages).
4. Immunological phenomena (such as glomerulonephritis or Osler's nodes).
5. Other microbiological evidence (such as a positive blood culture not matching a major criterion).

Two major criteria, or one major and three minor criteria, or all five minor criteria, are required to make a diagnosis of infective endocarditis.

In left-sided endocarditis, evidence of heart failure (such as pulmonary oedema), uncontrolled infection (such as fistula or pseudoaneurysms) or patients at high risk of embolism (such as a vegetation >10 mm with evidence of emboli despite antibiotics) would warrant early surgical intervention.

 KEY POINTS

- The clinical signs of aortic regurgitation are the result of a high-volume pulse which collapses in diastole.
- The presence of fever and a regurgitant murmur alone are not sufficient to make the diagnosis of endocarditis; the Duke criteria are an essential bedside tool for guiding clinical decision-making.
- Early discussion with the Cardiothoracic surgeons is suggested in decompensated patients.

CASE 42: EPISTAXIS

History

A 57-year-old woman is seen in the ENT clinic with recurrent epistaxis. She has no history of trauma, and is not anticoagulated, but states that she bruises easily.

Examination

On examination, she is 148 cm tall, and has a broad forehead with a short, webbed neck and widely spaced eyes. Her ears are low and rotated posteriorly, and she has subtle bilateral ptosis. She has a mid-line sternotomy scar and, on auscultation, she has a soft ejection systolic murmur appreciable at the upper right sternal border, with a loud second heart sound.

 INVESTIGATIONS

A full blood count and coagulation screen are normal.

? QUESTIONS

- Which syndrome is described here?
- What are the likely findings on echocardiogram?
- What are the non-cardiac manifestations of this condition?

ANSWER 42

Noonan syndrome is a genetic disorder with an autosomal dominant pattern of inheritance. Expression is variable, hence an affected parent is not always identified, and *de novo* mutations may also occur. Abnormalities in the *PTPN11* gene are most commonly implicated, which lead to attenuation of the RAS/MAPK cell signalling pathway. The differential diagnosis includes Turner's syndrome, however, Turner's only affects women and is associated with left-sided cardiac lesions. Other 'RASopathies', such as Costello syndrome, also present similar clinical findings to Noonan syndrome, but can be distinguished on genetic analysis.

The cardiac abnormalities associated with Noonan syndrome include pulmonary stenosis, atrial or ventricular septal defects and ventricular hypertrophy. Accordingly, this patient has evidence of a tissue pulmonary valve replacement, with a loud (but not metallic) second heart sound and an associated flow murmur. In cases of severe ventricular hypertrophy causing outflow tract obstruction, surgical septal myectomy may be necessary.

Pertinent to this case, non-cardiac manifestations include coagulopathy and platelet dysfunction, with the latter not necessarily evident on a full blood count. Partial deficiencies in factors VIII:C, XI:C and XII:C, as well as von Willebrand factor, have been reported. The typical facial characteristics are evident here; note that hypertelorism (widely spaced eyes) is almost ubiquitous in Noonan syndrome. A high-arched palate and micrognathia may also be found on closer examination. Skeletal defects, such as scoliosis, occur in about 30% and short stature may necessitate treatment with growth hormone. Intellectual development is variable; learning difficulties are not always present in Noonan syndrome.

 KEY POINTS

- Noonan syndrome is associated with congenital heart defects, most commonly pulmonary stenosis.
- Coagulopathy (or platelet dysfunction) is well-recognised as a non-cardiac manifestation.
- Inheritance is typically autosomal dominant although, due to variable expression, an affected parent is not always identified.

CASE 43: CHEST PAIN

History

A 66-year-old man presents with an 8-week history of recurrent central chest tightness, which occurs on strenuous exertion. The pain is relieved entirely by glyceryl trinitrate (GTN) spray within a few minutes. Regarding his past medical history, he underwent emergency percutaneous coronary intervention (PCI) to his left main stem and left anterior descending artery 2 years previously, with further staged PCI to his circumflex artery 6 months later. He is an ex-smoker.

He takes aspirin 75 mg, ticagrelor 60 mg twice daily, bisoprolol 10 mg, isosorbide mononitrate 20 mg twice daily, atorvastatin 40 mg, candesartan 16 mg, and nicorandil 20 mg twice daily.

Examination

His pulse is 55/min and his blood pressure is 92/62 mmHg. His heart sounds are normal and his chest is clear.

 INVESTIGATIONS

A myocardial perfusion scan is performed which shows a 5% burden of inducible ischaemia in the left ventricular anteroseptum. Ejection fraction remains preserved, and his 12-lead electrocardiogram (ECG) shows no new ischaemic changes.

? QUESTIONS

- What is the diagnosis?
- Should the patient be offered another angiogram?
- How could his medical treatment be optimised?

DOI: 10.1201/9781003350934-47

ANSWER 43

A constricting discomfort (or 'tightness') in the front of the chest, neck, shoulder or jaw, which is precipitated by physical exertion and relieved by rest (or GTN) fulfils the three criteria which constitute typical angina. Likewise, atypical angina meets two of these criteria, and a lone criterion suggests non-anginal chest pain.

In this case, the patient's symptoms are consistent with Canadian Cardiovascular Society (CCS) class I angina, in that they occur only on strenuous exertion. Given that a myocardial perfusion scan demonstrates a low (<10%) burden of ischaemia, it is reasonable to pursue medical management in the first instance. Whilst functional testing (such as a myocardial perfusion scan, stress magnetic resonance imaging [MRI] or stress echocardiogram) can be useful to identify the extent of any coronary perfusion defects, in patients with a high likelihood of obstructive coronary artery disease (such as this one) but with more severe symptoms despite medical therapy (e.g., CCS class III–IV), invasive angiogram could be offered directly.

This patient is already established on an extensive regimen of anti-anginals, including maximum beta blockade. His blood pressure is optimised and further increased dosages of vasodilators such as isosorbide mononitrate or nicorandil may therefore lead to symptomatic hypotension. Likewise, there is little room for additional heart rate control here. The introduction of ranolazine – which is believed to reduce myocardial oxygen demand via its action on sodium channels – may improve this patient's symptoms without altering his haemodynamic status.

In most patients who have undergone PCI, dual antiplatelet therapy is continued for 12 months, followed by lifelong aspirin therapy. Note that this patient remains on ticagrelor 60 mg twice daily, reduced from the usual 90 mg twice daily. This recommendation has been derived from the PEGASUS-TIMI 54 study, in which patients within 1 to 3 years of a myocardial infarction were continued on dual antiplatelet therapy for a median of 33 months and experienced fewer major adverse cardiovascular events (MACE) versus patients on aspirin alone. Extended dual antiplatelet therapy for up to 3 years may therefore be recommended in high-risk patients with myocardial infarction (such as those with PCI to their left main stem) who are not identified as having excessive bleeding risk.

 KEY POINTS

- History taking is essential in discerning whether chest pain is typical of angina.
- Even in patients with known coronary artery disease, in non-severe, stable angina, further optimisation of medical therapy is a reasonable first-line treatment strategy.
- Ranolazine is an option as an adjunctive antianginal drug and has negligible haemodynamic effects; it is initiated at a dose of 375 mg twice daily.

CASE 44: CARDIAC ARREST

History

A 29-year-old man collapses at a shopping centre. He is unresponsive and bystanders cannot find a pulse. They therefore commence cardiopulmonary resuscitation (CPR) and, upon the arrival of the paramedics, an external defibrillator is attached which shows ventricular fibrillation (VF). After a single 360 J shock, sustained return of spontaneous circulation is achieved. The patient is taken to the nearest emergency department conscious and alert.

Examination

On examination he is warm, with a normal radial pulse at 72/min. Blood pressure is 133/72 mmHg and oxygen saturations are 99% on air. He has tenderness over the sternum, however, heart sounds are normal and there is good air entry bilaterally.

🔎 **INVESTIGATIONS**

His 12-lead electrocardiogram (ECG) is shown in Figure 44.1.

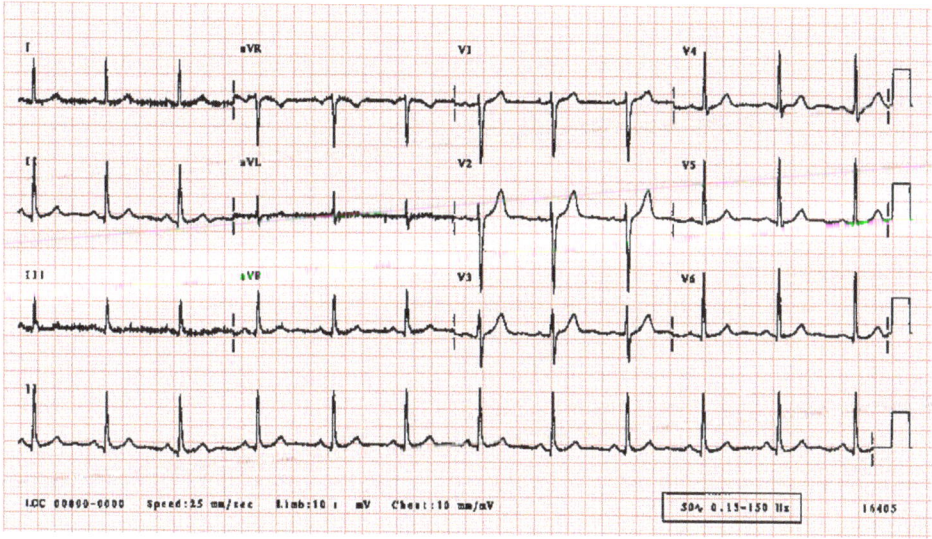

Figure 44.1 12-lead electrocardiogram.

Given his history of sudden cardiac arrest, an invasive coronary angiogram is performed, which demonstrates unobstructed coronary arteries, a normal ventriculogram and a normal aortogram. The patient is moved to the Coronary Care Unit (CCU) for cardiac monitoring.

❓ **QUESTIONS**

- What does the ECG show?
- What investigations should be performed?
- What is the most appropriate long-term management?

ANSWER 44

This patient's ECG is normal. Together with his normal coronary angiogram, acute coronary syndrome (ACS) can effectively be excluded as the cause of his VF arrest. There are subtypes of ACS in which coronary angiogram might be normal (such as protracted coronary spasm or thromboembolic events with spontaneous recanalisation of the artery), but these tend to be associated with ischaemic ECGs. Troponin is not a useful biomarker immediately after cardiac arrest and CPR, as cardiac injury is ubiquitous, so blood concentration will be elevated regardless of aetiology.

Extensive investigation is required here. Even with a normal ventriculogram, an underlying cardiomyopathy should be excluded in this age group. An echocardiogram uses ultrasound to examine heart muscle structure and function, together with the presence of any significant valvular lesions. In survivors of cardiac arrest, an echocardiogram may identify the increased ventricular volume in keeping with dilated cardiomyopathy or the asymmetrical hypertrophy (with or without outflow tract obstruction) pathognomonic of hypertrophic cardiomyopathy. However, the latter is usually detectable on ECG (which typically exhibits diffuse T wave inversion) and, hence, is an unlikely diagnosis in this case.

Whilst an echocardiogram is an accessible first-line imaging test, certain disease processes are undetectable with ultrasound alone. Gold standard functional and volumetric data, together with more detailed tissue characterisation, can be obtained using cardiac magnetic resonance imaging (MRI). Cardiac MRI can reveal areas of underlying scar or inflammation, such as in myocarditis which is a well-recognised cause of VF. Likewise, small patches of scarring may be evident in early cardiomyopathies such as in arrhythmogenic ventricular cardiomyopathy (AVC) – a common cause of ventricular arrhythmias in patients of this age.

In cases of documented VF where the heart is normal in structure, the prospect of an inherited arrhythmia should be addressed. In this patient's case, long QT syndrome seems unlikely based on his presenting ECG, however, in borderline cases, a treadmill test has the dual purpose of identifying appropriate QT shortening and excluding exercise-associated inherited arrhythmias, such as catecholaminergic polymorphic ventricular tachycardia (CPVT). Genetic testing to look for causative mutations associated with ventricular arrhythmias (such as in the *SCN5A* gene) can also help support the diagnosis of an inherited arrhythmia, however, results take several months to process.

For patients in whom VF can be clearly attributed to an ACS, provided full revascularisation is achieved, an implantable cardioverter-defibrillator (ICD) is not indicated. For all other cases of incapacitating ventricular arrhythmia, including apparently idiopathic VF, a secondary prevention ICD should be offered.

 KEY POINTS

- Ventricular fibrillation is most commonly seen during acute coronary syndromes.
- In the absence of causative coronary artery disease, inherited heart muscle conditions and inherited arrhythmias should be excluded.
- Cardiac MRI provides significant additive information over echocardiogram, including cases where the latter is normal.

Section 5
ENDOCRINOLOGY

CASE 45: WEIGHT GAIN

History

A 64-year-old man goes to his general practitioner (GP) because he has become increasingly overweight. He has gained 8 kg in weight over the past 6 months. He has noticed that he is constantly hungry and bruising easily. He finds it difficult to get up from his armchair or to climb stairs. He feels depressed and finds himself waking early in the mornings. He has had no previous physical or psychiatric illnesses. He is a retired miner and lives with his wife in a terraced house. He smokes 30 cigarettes per day and drinks 15 units of alcohol per week.

Examination

He is overweight, particularly in the abdominal region. There are purple stretch marks on his abdomen and thighs. His skin is thin and there are spontaneous bruises. His pulse is 76/min, regular and blood pressure is 168/104 mmHg. There is peripheral oedema. Otherwise, examination of his heart, respiratory and abdominal systems is normal. His neurological examination is otherwise normal, apart from some weakness in shoulder abduction and hip flexion.

🔍 INVESTIGATIONS

		Normal
Haemoglobin	13.2 g/dL	13.3–17.7 g/dL
Mean corpuscular volume (MCV)	87 fL	80–99 fL
White cell count	5.2 × 10⁹/L	3.9–10.6 × 10⁹/L
Platelets	237 × 10⁹/L	150–440 × 10⁹/L
Sodium	138 mmol/L	135–145 mmol/L
Potassium	3.3 mmol/L	3.5–5.0 mmol/L
Urea	6.2 mmol/L	2.5–6.7 mmol/L
Creatinine	113 µmol/L	70–120 µmol/L
Albumin	38 g/L	35–50 g/L
Glucose	8.3 mmol/L	4.0–6.0 mmol/L
Bilirubin	16 mmol/L	3–17 mmol/L
Alanine transaminase	24 IU/L	5–35 IU/L
Alkaline phosphatase	92 IU/L	30–300 IU/L
Gamma-glutamyl transpeptidase	43 IU/L	11–51 IU/L

Urinalysis: – protein; – blood; ++ glucose
Chest radiograph: normal

❓ QUESTIONS

- How would you investigate this patient?
- What is the likely diagnosis?
- How would you manage this patient?

ANSWER 45

The symptoms and signs of proximal myopathy, striae and truncal obesity are features of Cushing's syndrome. Fat accumulation causes a 'moon face', a 'buffalo hump' and enlarged fat pads in the supraclavicular fossae. The hyperglycaemia and hypokalaemia would fit this diagnosis. In addition, psychiatric disturbances, typically depression, may occur in Cushing's syndrome. Cushing's disease is due to a pituitary adenoma secreting adrenocorticotrophic hormone (ACTH). The term *Cushing's syndrome* is a wider one and encompasses a group of disorders caused by overproduction of cortisol.

> **! CAUSES OF CUSHING'S SYNDROME**
>
> - ACTH secretion by a basophil adenoma of the anterior pituitary gland (Cushing's disease).
> - Ectopic ACTH secretion (e.g., from a bronchial carcinoma), often causing a massive release of cortisol and a severe and rapid onset of symptoms.
> - Primary adenoma/carcinoma of the adrenal cortex (suppressed ACTH).
> - Iatrogenic: Corticosteroid treatment. This is the commonest cause in day-to-day clinical practice.

This patient's primary presenting complaint is rapid-onset obesity. The principal causes of obesity are:

- Genetic
- Environmental: Excessive food intake, lack of exercise
- Hormonal:
  - Hypothyroidism
  - Cushing's syndrome
  - Polycystic ovaries and hyperprolactinaemia
- Alcohol-induced pseudo-Cushing's syndrome

This patient should be investigated by an endocrinologist. The first point is to establish that this man has abnormal cortisol secretion. There should be loss of the normal diurnal rhythm with an elevated midnight cortisol level or increased urinary conjugated cortisol excretion. A dexamethasone suppression test would normally suppress cortisol excretion. It is then important to exclude common causes of abnormal cortisol excretion, such as stress/depression or alcohol abuse. Measurement of ACTH levels distinguishes between adrenal (low ACTH) and pituitary/ectopic (high ACTH) causes. This patient drinks alcohol moderately and has a normal gamma-glutamyl transpeptidase. His depression seems to be a consequence of his cortisol excess rather than a cause, as he has no psychiatric history.

His ACTH level is elevated. Bronchial carcinoma is a possibility as he is a heavy smoker, and the onset of his Cushing's syndrome has been rapid. However, his chest radiograph is normal. In this man, a magnetic resonance imaging (MRI) scan (T1-weighted coronal image) through the pituitary shows a hypointense microadenoma (Figure 45.1, arrow). This can be treated with surgery or radiotherapy. Trans-sphenoidal microadenomectomy is the treatment of choice as it cures the patient and leaves them with normal hypothalamic–pituitary–adrenal function.

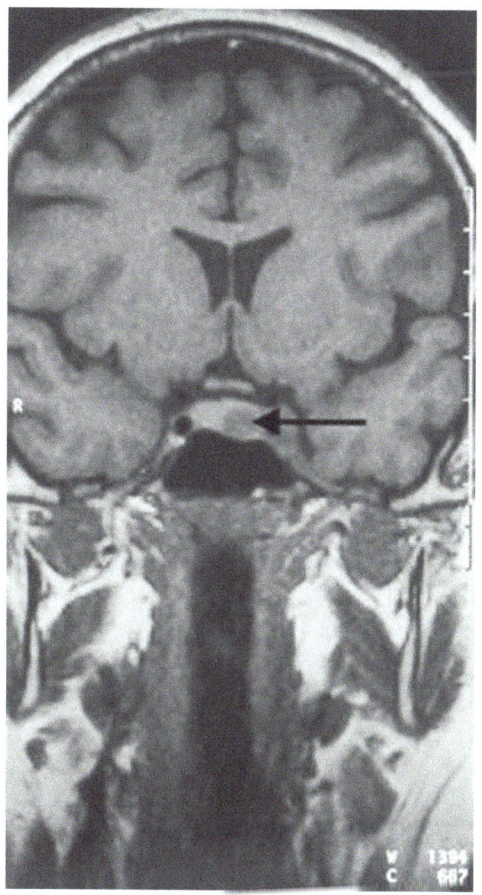

Figure 45.1 Magnetic resonance imaging scan through the pituitary.

🔑 **KEY POINTS**

- Patients with rapid-onset obesity should have endocrine causes excluded.
- Corticosteroid treatment is the commonest cause for Cushing's syndrome.
- Patients with severe and rapid-onset Cushing's syndrome often have ectopic ACTH secretion or cortisol-secreting adrenal tumours.

CASE 46: TIREDNESS

History

A 55-year-old man presents to his general practitioner (GP) complaining of lack of energy. He has become increasingly tired over the past 18 months. He works as a solicitor and describes episodes when he has fallen asleep in his office. He is unable to stay awake after 9:30 pm and sleeps through until 7:30 am. He finds it difficult to concentrate at work and has stopped playing his weekly game of tennis. He had an episode of depression 10 years ago related to the break-up of his first marriage. He has no current personal problems. He has had no other major illnesses. His brother developed type 1 diabetes mellitus at the age of 13. On direct questioning, he has noticed that he has become more constipated but denies any abdominal pain or rectal bleeding. He has put on 8 kg in weight over the past year.

Examination

On examination, he is overweight. His facial skin is dry and scaly. His pulse is 56/min, regular and blood pressure is 146/88 mmHg. Examination of his cardiovascular, respiratory and abdominal systems is unremarkable. Neurological examination showed a little proximal weakness.

🔍 INVESTIGATIONS

		Normal
Haemoglobin	11.8 g/dL	13.3–17.7 g/dL
Mean corpuscular volume (MCV)	96 fL	80–99 fL
White cell count	4.3×10^9/L	$3.9–10.6 \times 10^9$/L
Platelets	154×10^9/L	$150–440 \times 10^9$/L
Sodium	140 mmol/L	135–145 mmol/L
Potassium	4.4 mmol/L	3.5–5.0 mmol/L
Urea	6.4 mmol/L	2.5–6.7 mmol
Creatinine	125 µmol/L	70–120 µmol/L
Glucose	4.7 mmol/L	4.0–6.0 mmol/L
Calcium	2.48 mmol/L	2.12–2.65 mmol/L
Phosphate	1.20 mmol/L	0.8–1.45 mmol/L
Cholesterol	6.4 mmol/L	3.9–6.0 mmol/L
Triglycerides	1.4 mmol/L	0.55–1.90 mmol/L

Urinalysis: nothing abnormal detected (NAD)

❓ QUESTIONS

- What is the likely diagnosis?
- How would you further examine and investigate this patient?
- How would you manage this patient?

DOI: 10.1201/9781003350934-51

ANSWER 46

Fatigue is a very common symptom of both physical and mental illness. The differential diagnosis is extensive and includes cancer, depression, anaemia, renal failure and endocrine diseases. In this case, the main differentials are depression and hypothyroidism. He has a history of depression but currently has no obvious triggers for a further episode of depression. He is not waking early in the morning or having difficulty getting to sleep, which are common biological symptoms of severe depression. There are a number of clues in this case to the diagnosis of hypothyroidism. Insidious onset of fatigue, difficulty concentrating, increased somnolence, constipation and weight gain are features of hypothyroidism. As in this case, there may be a family or past medical history of other autoimmune diseases such as type 1 diabetes mellitus, vitiligo or Addison's disease. Hypothyroidism typically presents in the fifth or sixth decade and is about five times more common in women than men. Obstructive sleep apnoea is associated with hypothyroidism and may contribute to daytime sleepiness and fatigue.

On examination, the facial appearances and bradycardia are consistent with the diagnosis. Characteristically, patients with overt hypothyroidism have dry, scaly, cold and thickened skin. There may be a malar flush against the background of the pale facial appearance (*strawberries-and-cream appearance*). Scalp hair is usually brittle and sparse, and there may be thinning of the lateral third of the eyebrows. Bradycardia may occur, and the apex beat may be difficult to locate because of the presence of a pericardial effusion. A classic sign of hypothyroidism is the delayed relaxation phase of the ankle jerk. Other neurological syndromes that may occur in association with hypothyroidism include carpal tunnel syndrome, proximal muscle weakness, a cerebellar syndrome or polyneuritis. Patients may present with psychiatric illnesses, including psychoses (*myxoedema madness*).

Clues to the diagnosis in the investigations are the mild normochromic, normocytic anaemia, marginally raised creatinine and hypercholesterolaemia. The anaemia of hypothyroidism is typically normochromic, normocytic or macrocytic; microcytic anaemia may occur if there is menorrhagia. A macrocytic anaemia may represent undiagnosed vitamin B_{12} deficiency. Renal blood flow is reduced in hypothyroidism, and this can cause the creatinine to be slightly above the normal range.

The most severe cases of hypothyroidism present with myxoedema coma, with bradycardia, reduced respiratory rate and severe hypothermia. Typically, shivering is absent.

In this case, the thyroid function tests showed thyroid-stimulating hormone (TSH), 73 mU/L (normal range <6 mU/L); free thyroxine (T4), 3 pmol/L (normal range 9–22 pmol/L). The high TSH indicates primary hypothyroidism rather than hypopituitarism. The commonest cause of hypothyroidism is autoimmune thyroiditis, and the patient should have thyroid peroxidase (TPO) autoantibodies assayed.

!   **CAUSES OF HYPOTHYROIDISM**

- Autoimmune thyroiditis
- Subacute thyroiditis (de Quervain's)
- Post-thyroidectomy
- Post-radioiodine treatment for thyrotoxicosis
- Drugs for treatment of hyperthyroidism: Carbimazole, propylthiouracil
- Amiodarone, lithium
- Dietary iodine deficiency
- Inherited enzyme defects
- Panhypopituitarism
- Genetic conditions such as Down syndrome, Turner's syndrome

Treatment is with T4 at a maintenance dose of 75–200 μg/day. Response is measured clinically and biochemically by the return of TSH to the normal range. NICE guidelines recommend starting levothyroxine with 1.6 μg/kg/day for patients under age 65 and no history of cardiovascular disease. Elderly patients or those with coronary heart disease should be started cautiously on T4 because of the risk of precipitating myocardial ischaemia. In existing hypothyroidism of female patients who become pregnant, dosing of thyroxine should be increased by at least 25–50 μg along with regular TSH monitoring. Common side effects of thyroxine replacement include hyperthyroidism, atrial fibrillation, aggravating angina and osteopenia. Liothyronine, either alone or in combination with levothyroxine, is not offered routinely for hypothyroidism patients as the long-term effects are uncertain.

 KEY POINTS

- Hypothyroidism should be considered in the differential diagnosis of any patient presenting with fatigue.
- A neurological examination should be part of the routine assessment of all such patients.
- Clinical symptoms of hypothyroidism are usually non-specific.
- Hypothyroidism may present in unusual ways, such as psychoses or decreased consciousness level.
- Autoimmune thyroiditis is the commonest cause of hypothyroidism.

CASE 47: THIRST AND FREQUENCY

History

A 63-year-old woman is referred to a nephrologist for investigation of polyuria. About 4 weeks ago, she developed abrupt-onset extreme thirst and polyuria. She is getting up to pass urine five times a night. Over the past 3 months, she has felt generally unwell and noted pain in her back. She has lost 3 kg in weight over this time. She also has a persistent frontal headache associated with early morning nausea. The headache is worsened by coughing or lying down. Eight years previously, she had a left mastectomy and radiotherapy for carcinoma of the breast. She is a retired civil servant who is a non-smoker and drinks 10 units of alcohol per week. She is on no medication.

Examination

She is thin and her muscles are wasted. Her pulse rate is 72/min, blood pressure is 120/84 mmHg, jugular venous pressure is not raised, heart sounds are normal and she has no peripheral oedema. Examination of her respiratory, abdominal and neurological systems is normal. Her fundi show papilloedema.

🔍 INVESTIGATIONS

		Normal
Haemoglobin	12.2 g/dL	11.7–15.7 g/dL
Mean corpuscular volume (MCV)	85 fL	80–99 fL
White cell count	6.7×10^9/L	$3.5–11.0 \times 10^9$/L
Platelets	312×10^9/L	$150–440 \times 10^9$/L
Sodium	142 mmol/L	135–145 mmol/L
Potassium	3.8 mmol/L	3.5–5.0 mmol/L
Bicarbonate	26 mmol/L	24–30 mmol/L
Urea	4.2 mmol/L	2.5–6.7 mmol/L
Creatinine	68 µmol/L	70–120 µmol/L
Glucose	4.2 mmol/L	4.0–6.0 mmol/L
Albumin	38 g/L	35–50 g/L
Calcium	2.75 mmol/L	2.12–2.65 mmol/L
Phosphate	1.2 mmol/L	0.8–1.45 mmol/L
Bilirubin	12 mmol/L	3–17 mmol/L
Alanine transaminase	35 IU/L	5–35 IU/L
Alkaline phosphatase	690 IU/L	30–300 IU/L

Urinalysis: no protein; no blood

❓ QUESTIONS

- What is the likely cause of her polyuria?
- How would you investigate this patient?
- How would you manage this patient?

ANSWER 47

Polyuria is generally defined as a urine output >3 litres a day in adults. True polyuria must be distinguished from frequency and nocturia, which are generally due to bladder or prostate conditions.

This woman has mild hypercalcaemia, but this is not high enough to explain her extreme thirst and polyuria. It is more likely that she has polyuria due to neurogenic or central diabetes insipidus as a result of secondary metastases in her hypothalamus. The hypercalcaemia and raised alkaline phosphatase are suggestive of bony metastases secondary to her breast cancer. The recent-onset headache, worsened by coughing and lying down and associated with vomiting, is characteristic of raised intracranial pressure, which is confirmed by the presence of papilloedema. If there is a lesion around the pituitary, there may be compression of the optic nerve, causing visual field abnormalities. Absent glycosuria in urinalysis and normal serum glucose levels rules out diabetes mellitus as a cause of polyuria.

Neurogenic diabetes insipidus is due to inadequate arginine vasopressin (AVP) secretion. About 30% of cases are idiopathic. The remaining causes are neoplastic, infectious, inflammatory (granulomas), traumatic (neurosurgery, injury) or vascular (cerebral haemorrhage, infarction). Patients typically describe an abrupt onset of polyuria and polydipsia. This is because urinary concentration can be maintained fairly well until the number of AVP-secreting neurons in the hypothalamus decreases to 10–15% of the normal number, after which AVP levels decrease to a range where urine output increases dramatically.

! MAJOR CAUSES OF POLYURIA AND POLYDIPSIA

- Solute diuresis (e.g., diabetes mellitus)
- Renal diseases that impair urinary concentrating mechanisms (e.g., chronic renal failure)
- Drinking abnormalities: Psychogenic polydipsia
- Renal resistance to the action of AVP
- Nephrogenic diabetes insipidus (due to inherited defects in either the AVP V_2 receptor or the aquaporin-2 receptor)
- Hypokalaemia
- Hypercalcaemia
- Drugs (e.g., lithium, demeclocycline)

A water-deprivation test could be performed in this patient, measuring the plasma sodium, urine volume and urine osmolality until the sodium rises above 146 mmol/L, or the urine osmolality reaches a plateau and the patient has lost at least 2% of body weight. At this point, AVP is measured and the response to subcutaneous desmopressin is measured. An increase in urine osmolality >50% indicates central diabetes insipidus and <10% nephrogenic diabetes insipidus. The hypothalamus should be imaged by magnetic resonance imaging (MRI) scanning and bone radiographs and bone scans should be performed to identify metastases. The MRI scan (T_1-weighted coronal image) through the pituitary in Figure 47.1 shows thickening of the pituitary stalk due to metastatic disease (left arrow) and partial replacement of the normal bone marrow of the clivus by metastatic tumour (right arrow). Treatment of neurogenic diabetes insipidus involves a regular DDAVP (l-deamino-8-d-arginine vasopressin) dose titrated to treatment response. To reduce ongoing symptoms and for treatment maintenance, conservative management includes avoiding rapid overcorrection of hypernatremia, regular fluid status assessment, fluid replacement, strict adherence to desmopressin requirements and monitoring serum sodium levels. She should be referred to an oncologist for treatment of her metastatic carcinoma.

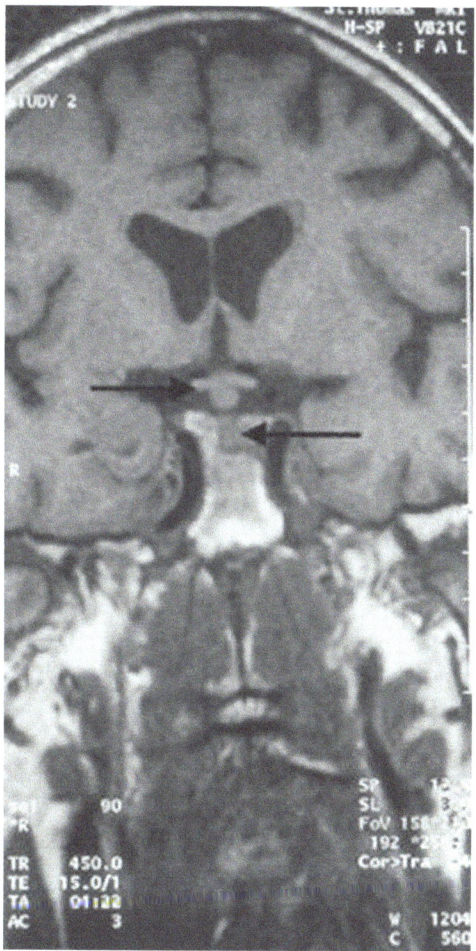

Figure 47.1 Magnetic resonance imaging scan through the pituitary.

🔑 **KEY POINTS**

- The commonest causes of polyuria are diabetes mellitus and chronic renal failure.
- True polyuria must be distinguished from frequency and nocturia due to lower urinary tract pathology.
- Breast carcinoma may recur after several years of remission.

History

A 72-year-old woman develops a chest infection and is treated at home with doxycycline by her general practitioner (GP). She lives alone, but one of her daughters, a retired nurse, moves in to look after her. The patient has a long history of rheumatoid arthritis, which is still active and for which she has taken 7 mg of prednisolone daily for 9 years. She takes paracetamol occasionally for joint pain. There is no other relevant past or family history. When the GP visited, he found her blood pressure to be 138/82 mmHg.

For 5 days, she has been feverish and anorexic and confined to bed. Her daughter has made her drink plenty of fluids. On the fifth day, she became drowsy and her daughter had increasing difficulty in rousing her, so she called an ambulance to take her to the emergency department.

Examination

She is small (assessed as 50 kg), but there is no evidence of recent weight loss. Her temperature is 38.8°C. She is drowsy and responds to commands but will not answer simple questions. There is a global reduction in muscle tone but no focal neurological signs. Her pulse is 118/min, blood pressure is 104/68 mmHg and the jugular venous pressure is not raised. There is no ankle swelling. In the chest, there are bilateral basal crackles and wheezes. Her joints show slight active inflammation and deformity, in keeping with the history of rheumatoid arthritis.

🔎 INVESTIGATIONS

		Normal
Haemoglobin	11.5 g/dL	11.7–15.7 g/dL
Mean corpuscular volume (MCV)	86 fL	80–99 fL
White cell count	13.2 × 10⁹/L	3.5–11.0 × 10⁹/L
Platelets	376 × 10⁹/L	150–440 × 10⁹/L
Sodium	125 mmol/L	135–145 mmol/L
Potassium	4.7 mmol/L	3.5–5.0 mmol/L
Urea	8.4 mmol/L	2.5–6.7 mmol/L
Creatinine	131 µmol/L	70–120 µmol/L
Glucose	4.8 mmol/L	4.0–6.0 mmol/L

? QUESTIONS

- What is the diagnosis?
- How would you explain the abnormal investigations?
- How would you manage this case?

DOI: 10.1201/9781003350934-53

ANSWER 48

The likeliest diagnosis is secondary acute hypoaldosteronism due to failure of the hypothalamic–pituitary–adrenal axis caused by the long-term prednisolone use. This is a common problem in patients on long-term steroids and arises when there is a need for increased glucocorticoid output, most frequently seen in infections or trauma, including surgery, or when the patient has prolonged vomiting and, therefore, cannot take the oral steroid effectively. It presents as here with drowsiness and low blood pressure.

The hyponatraemia is another result of the superimposed illness. It is probably due to a combination of reduced intake of sodium, owing to the anorexia, and dilution of plasma by the fluid intake. In secondary hypoaldosteronism, the renin–angiotensin–aldosterone system is intact and should operate to retain sodium. This is in contrast to acute primary hypoaldosteronism (*Addisonian crisis*), when the mineralocorticoid secretion fails as well as the glucocorticoid secretion, causing hyponatraemia and hyperkalaemia. Acute secondary hypoaldosteronism is often, but erroneously, called an Addisonian crisis.

Spread of the infection should also be considered with the prime sites being to the brain, with either meningitis or cerebral abscess, or locally to cause a pulmonary abscess or empyema. The patient has a degree of immunosuppression due to her age and the long-term steroid use. The dose of steroid is higher than may appear at first sight as the patient is only 50 kg; drug doses are usually denoted for a 70 kg male, which in this case would equate to 10 mg of prednisolone, that is, an increase of 40% on her dose of 7 mg.

The treatment is immediate empirical intravenous infusion of hydrocortisone, usually 100 mg IV/IM stat (then every 6 hours until patient is stabilised), IV normal saline (1 litre over 30–60 minutes) or IV dextrose if hypoglycaemic, regular blood glucose check and treat hypoglycaemia if present. The patient responded and, in 5 h, her consciousness level was normal and her blood pressure had risen to 136/78 mmHg. Chest radiograph showed bilateral shadowing consistent with pneumonia, but no other abnormality.

 KEY POINTS

- Secondary hypoaldosteronism is a medical emergency and requires immediate empirical treatment.
- Patients on long-term steroids should have the dose increased when they have intercurrent illnesses and replaced systemically when they have persistent vomiting.

History

A 33-year-old housewife has noticed that she is becoming tired and having difficulty coping with her two children, aged 6 and 4 years. She goes to see her general practitioner (GP) because she feels she may be suffering from anxiety and depression. She felt more irritable and anxious than usual. Her sleep and appetite have been normal, but she has lost some weight. Her change in personality has been noticed by her husband and friends. She feels constantly restless and has difficulty concentrating on a subject for more than a few moments. Her increased anxiety has developed over the past 3 months. She has also noticed an increased frequency of bowel movements. Her periods have become lighter and shorter. She feels extremely tired and thinks that she has been prone to sweat more than usual. She has had no significant illnesses previously. She is a non-smoker and drinks 10 units of alcohol per week.

Examination

She appears agitated and her hands are sweaty and tremulous. Her pulse is 104/min and regular; her blood pressure is 130/70 mmHg. Her proximal muscles seem a little weak. There are no abnormalities in the cardiovascular, respiratory, abdominal or nervous systems. Investigations are organised by her GP.

INVESTIGATIONS		
		Normal
Haemoglobin	13.3 g/dL	11.7–15.7 g/dL
White cell count	4.7×10^9/L	$3.5–11.0 \times 10^9$/L
Platelets	246×10^9/L	$150–440 \times 10^9$/L
Sodium	142 mmol/L	135–145 mmol/L
Potassium	4.6 mmol/L	3.5–5.0 mmol/L
Bicarbonate	22 mmol/L	24–30 mmol/L
Urea	5.2 mmol/L	2.5–6.7 mmol/L
Creatinine	78 µmol/L	70–120 µmol/L
Glucose	4.2 mmol/L	4.0–6.0 mmol/L

Urinalysis: no blood; no protein

? QUESTIONS

- What is the most likely diagnosis?
- What examination and investigation would you do for this patient?
- How would you manage this patient?

ANSWER 49

Although anxiety might produce some of these symptoms and signs, they fit much better with a diagnosis of hyperthyroidism. The neck should be examined carefully and, in this case, there was a smooth goitre with no bruit over it. Blood tests showed a very low thyroxine-stimulating hormone (TSH) level and high free thyroxine (T4), confirming the diagnosis of hyperthyroidism due to a diffuse toxic goitre (Graves' disease). Hyperthyroidism may mimic an anxiety neurosis with marked restlessness, irritability and distraction. The most helpful discriminatory symptoms are weight loss despite a normal appetite and preference for cold weather. The most helpful signs are goitre, especially with a bruit audible over it, resting sinus tachycardia or atrial fibrillation, tremor and eye signs. Eye signs that may be present include lid retraction (sclera visible below the upper lid), lid lag, proptosis, oedema of the eyelids, congestion of the conjunctiva and ophthalmoplegia. Atypical presentations of thyrotoxicosis include atrial fibrillation in younger patients, unexplained weight loss, proximal myopathy or a toxic confusional state. The weakness here is suggestive of a proximal myopathy. The very low TSH level indicates a primary thyroid disease rather than the far less common overproduction of TSH by the anterior pituitary.

! COMMON CAUSES OF HYPERTHYROIDISM

- Diffuse toxic goitre (Graves' disease)
- Toxic nodular goitre
  - Multinodular goitre (Plummer's disease)
  - Solitary toxic adenoma
- Over-replacement with thyroxine
- Postpartum thyroiditis
- Amiodarone therapy

Blood should be sent for thyroid-stimulating immunoglobulin, which will be detected in patients with Graves' disease. Medical treatment for thyrotoxicosis involves the use of the antithyroid drugs such as carbimazole or propylthiouracil. These are given for 12–18 months, but there is a 50% chance of disease recurrence on stopping the drugs. If this happens, radioiodine or surgery is indicated. Beta-blockers can be used to rapidly improve the symptoms of sympathetic overactivity (tachycardia, tremor) while waiting for the antithyroid drugs to act. Radioiodine is effective, but there is a high incidence of late hypothyroidism. Contraindications to radioiodine treatment include pregnancy and thyroid eye disease. Surgery is indicated if medical treatment fails or if the gland is large and compressing surrounding structures. In severe exophthalmos, there is a risk of corneal damage and ophthalmological advice should be sought. High-dose steroids, lateral tarsorrhaphy or orbital decompression may be needed.

🔑 KEY POINTS

- Thyrotoxicosis may be difficult to differentiate from an anxiety state. In older patients, symptoms such as palpitations, breathlessness and oedema may predominate.
- The commonest causes of hyperthyroidism are Graves' disease or a toxic nodular goitre.

CASE 50: LOSS OF CONSCIOUSNESS

History

A 40-year-old man is admitted to the emergency department having been found unconscious at home by his wife on her return from work in the evening. He has suffered from insulin-dependent diabetes mellitus for 24 years, and his diabetic control is poor. He has had recurrent hypoglycaemic episodes and has been treated in the emergency department on two occasions for this. Over the past few weeks, he has developed pain in his right foot. His general practitioner diagnosed cellulitis, and he has received two courses of oral antibiotics. This has made him feel unwell, and he has complained to his wife of fatigue and anorexia and feeling thirsty. In his medical history, he had a myocardial infarction 2 years ago. He has had bilateral laser treatment for proliferative diabetic retinopathy. He was a builder but is now unemployed. He smokes 25 cigarettes per week and drinks around 30 units of alcohol per week. His treatment is twice-daily insulin; he checks his blood glucose irregularly at home.

Examination

He looks dry with reduced skin turgor and poor capillary return. His pulse is regular and 116/min. His blood pressure is 98/72 mmHg lying, 74/50 mmHg sitting up. He seems short of breath, with a respiratory rate of 30/min. Otherwise, examination of his respiratory and abdominal systems is normal. He has an ulcer on the third toe of his right foot, and the foot looks red and feels warm. He is rousable only to painful stimuli. There is no focal neurology. Fundoscopy shows bilateral scars of laser therapy.

🔍 INVESTIGATIONS

		Normal
Haemoglobin	15.? g/dL	11.7–15.7 g/dL
White cell count	16.3 × 10⁹/L	3.5–11.0 × 10⁹/L
Platelets	344 × 10⁹/L	150–440 × 10⁹/L
Sodium	143 mmol/L	135–145 mmol/L
Potassium	5.5 mmol/L	3.5–5.0 mmol/L
Chloride	105 mmol/l	95–105 mmol/L
Urea	11.3 mmol/L	2.5–6.7 mmol/L
Creatinine	114 µmol/L	70–120 µmol/L
Bicarbonate	12 mmol/L	24–30 mmol/L

Urinalysis: ++ protein; ++ ketones; +++ glucose
Blood gases on air

pH	7.27	7.38–7.44
$PaCO_2$	3.0 kPa	4.7–6.0 kPa
p_aO_2	13.4 kPa	12.0–14.5 kP

❓ QUESTIONS

- What are the differential diagnoses for this patient?
- What is the cause for this patient's coma?
- How would you manage this patient?

ANSWER 50

This man has signs of dehydration and the high urea with a normal creatinine is consistent with this. He is acidotic. The blood glucose level is not given, but the picture is likely to represent hyperglycaemic ketoacidotic coma. The key clinical features on examination are dehydration shown by skin signs, significant postural hypotension and hyperventilation secondary to a metabolic acidosis and the triggering problem with the infection in the foot. A persistently high glucose level induced by the response to an infected foot ulcer causes heavy glycosuria, triggering an osmotic diuresis. This leads to hypovolaemia and reduced renal blood flow, causing prerenal uraemia. The extracellular hyperosmolality causes severe cellular dehydration, and loss of water from his brain cells is the cause of his coma. Decreased insulin activity with intracellular glucose deficiency stimulates lipolysis and the production of ketoacids. He has a high anion gap metabolic acidosis due to accumulation of ketoacids (acetoacetate and 3-hydroxybutyrate). The anion gap is calculated from the following equation:

$$[Na^+]+[K^+]-([Cl^-]+[HCO_3^-])$$

It is normally 10–18 mmol/L; in this case it is 31.5 mmol/L. Ketones cause a characteristically sickly sweet smell on the breath of patients with diabetic ketoacidosis (about 20% of the population cannot smell the ketones). The metabolic acidosis stimulates the respiratory centre, leading to an increase in the rate and depth of respiration (Kussmaul breathing) and producing the reduction in $PaCO_2$ as respiratory compensation for the acidosis. In older diabetic patients, there is often evidence of infection (e.g., bronchopneumonia, infected foot ulcer) precipitating these metabolic abnormalities.

The differential diagnosis of coma in diabetics includes non-ketotic hyperglycaemic coma, particularly in elderly diabetics; lactic acidosis, especially in patients on metformin; profound hypoglycaemia; and non-metabolic causes for coma (e.g., cerebrovascular attacks and drug overdose). Salicylate poisoning may cause hyperglycaemia, hyperventilation and coma, but the metabolic picture is usually one of dominant respiratory alkalosis and mild metabolic acidosis.

The aims of management are to correct the massive fluid and electrolyte losses, hyperglycaemia and metabolic acidosis. Rapid fluid replacement with intravenous normal saline and potassium supplements should be started. In younger patients, a slower infusion rate may be indicated as common complications due to incorrect fluid therapy lead to cerebral oedema. In patients with cardiac or renal disease, a central venous pressure (CVP) line is needed to control fluid balance. Regular monitoring of plasma potassium is essential, as it may fall very rapidly as glucose enters cells. Insulin therapy (0.1 unit/kg/hour) is given by intravenous infusion adjusted according to blood glucose levels. Patients already on long-acting insulin should be continued. Short-acting insulin should be withheld. A nasogastric tube is used to prevent aspiration of gastric contents and a bladder catheter is needed to measure urine production. Antibiotics and local wound care should be given to treat this man's foot ulcer. In the longer term, it is important that this patient and his wife are educated about his diabetes and that he has regular access to diabetes services. His smoking and alcohol consumption will also need to be addressed. There may be social issues to be considered in relation to his unemployment.

🔑 **KEY POINTS**

- Dehydration, tachypnoea and ketosis are the key clinical signs of diabetic ketoacidosis.
- Twenty percent of the population (and therefore doctors) cannot smell ketones.

CASE 51: NUMB FEET

History

A 66-year-old man presents with numb feet. In the last few months, his feet have felt as though he is wearing thick socks and his feet burn at night. He recently cut his foot whilst walking barefoot in the back garden and didn't feel any pain. He has also been thirstier than usual and has been drinking soft drinks to slake his thirst.

He had an inguinal hernia repaired 2 years ago and he stopped smoking then on the advice of the anaesthetist. Previously, he smoked 20 cigarettes per day. He drinks 4 pints of beer on weekends. His father died of a myocardial infarction at age 58.

Examination

His blood pressure is 136/84 mmHg. The respiratory, cardiovascular and abdominal systems are normal. There is a 3 cm ulcerated area with a well-demarcated edge on the dorsum of the right foot. The posterior tibial pulses and dorsalis pedis pulses are palpable. The capillary return time is 2 seconds. The neurological examination reveals loss of light touch, vibration and pinprick sensation to the ankles. Power in the feet, legs and hands is normal. Ankle jerk is absent bilaterally. Plantar reflexes are down going. There is some loss of pinprick sensation in the hands. The rest of the neurological examination is normal.

INVESTIGATIONS		
		Normal
Haemoglobin	14.3 g/dL	13.7–17.7 g/dL
White cell count	7.4 × 10⁹/L	3.9–10.6 × 10⁹/L
Neutrophils	4.6 × 10⁹/L	1.8–7.7 × 10⁹/L
Lymphocytes	2.5 × 10⁹/L	0.6–4.8 × 10⁹/L
Platelets	372 × 10⁹/L	150–440 × 10⁹/L
Sodium	140 mmol/L	135–145 mmol/L
Potassium	4.0 mmol/L	3.5–5.0 mmol/L
Urea	5.1 mmol/L	2.5–6.7 mmol/L
Creatinine	89 µmol/L	70–120 µmol/L
Glucose	12.4 mmol/L	4.0–6.0 mmol/L
HbA$_{1c}$	9.1%	<7%

? QUESTIONS

- What is the likely diagnosis?
- What further investigations should be carried out?
- What is the management for this patient?

DOI: 10.1201/9781003350934-56

ANSWER 51

The glove and stocking distribution of sensory loss with preservation of motor power suggests a peripheral sensory neuropathy. Causes of a peripheral neuropathy are listed in Table 51.1. The raised HbA_{1c} suggests diabetes and prolonged hyperglycaemia.

Peripheral neuropathy may be the first sign of type 2 diabetes mellitus. Initially, sensory loss can be subtle, usually with loss of ankle jerks and vibration in the feet. Subclinical neuropathy can be detected using a monofilament. As the neuropathy progresses, pinprick sensation is lost and the hands may be involved. In later stages, foot deformity can occur. Charcot (neuropathic) joint is caused by repeated joint injury due to the loss of pain sensation. Diabetic neuropathy may lead to unrecognised trauma to the skin, which then heals poorly. Diabetic neuropathy and peripheral vascular disease often co-exist and can lead to gangrene.

Further investigations in this patient should include vitamin B_{12} and folate level, thyroid function, erythrocyte sedimentation rate (ESR), protein electrophoresis, ANCA and ANA. Genetic tests for an inherited neuropathy or a lead level might be considered if there is a suspicion for these conditions. Alcohol abuse should be apparent from the history, but a reduced red blood cell ketolase level can be used to confirm vitamin B1 (thiamine) deficiency. In diabetic neuropathy, nerve conduction studies are rarely needed, but may be helpful to exclude an entrapment neuropathy such as carpel tunnel syndrome. Co-existing peripheral vascular disease is common in diabetes and measurement of the ankle: brachial blood pressure ratio should be performed if there are absent lower limb pulses. A value less than 0.97 suggests arterial disease. The development of one diabetic complication should prompt the search for other complications: diabetic retinopathy, nephropathy, coronary and carotid vascular disease.

Treatment of type 2 diabetes mellitus includes dietary advice, oral hypoglycaemics and possibly insulin. The goal is for a HbA_{1c} less than 7.5%. Blood glucose control can slow progression of diabetic neuropathy. Prevention of diabetic foot ulcers is essential and should include use of comfortable shoes, avoiding bare feet, regular chiropody and aggressive treatment of nail infections. Diabetic neuropathy that is painful may benefit from amitriptyline, gabapentin or topical capsaicin cream. Antibiotics and specialist dressings may be required if foot

TABLE 51.1 Causes of peripheral neuropathy

- Diabetes mellitus
- Carcinoma
- Critical illness
- Drugs (including amiodarone, cisplatin, isoniazid, metronidazole, nitrofurantoin, vincristine)
- Toxins (alcohol, arsenic, lead, thallium)
- Genetic (Charcot–Marie–Tooth disease, Fabry's disease, Friedrich's ataxia)
- Vitamin deficiencies (vitamin B1-thiamine, vitamin B3-niacin, vitamin B6-pyrodoxine, vitamin B_{12}-cyanocobalamin)
- Uraemia
- Chronic liver disease
- Human immunodeficiency virus (HIV)
- Lymphoma
- Multiple myeloma
- Benign monoclonal gammopathy
- Primary systemic amyloidosis

ulcers develop. Osteomyelitis is common in deep ulcers for which **MRI** is the investigation of choice. Regular follow-up of patients with type 2 diabetes to prevent foot disease should include neurological and vascular examination of both feet and testing for peripheral neuropathy with a monofilament.

 KEY POINTS

- Peripheral neuropathy maybe the first presentation of type 2 diabetes mellitus.
- Diabetic feet are particularly vulnerable because of sensory loss, arterial insufficiency and high sugars.

CASE 52: CHANGE IN CHARACTER

History

A 66-year-old man has been persuaded by his wife to go to his general practitioner (GP). She is worried that he has changed. Over the last 4 weeks he has become lethargic and rather vague. He has a 12-year history of chronic cough and sputum production, but she thinks that these symptoms may have increased a little over the last 8 weeks. He has smoked 20 cigarettes daily for the last 50 years, and he drinks about 14 units of alcohol per week. Two years ago, he became depressed and was treated with an antidepressant for 6 months with good effect. She cannot remember the name of the medication. He had worked all his life as a postman until retirement 6 years ago.

Examination

He is a little vague in his answers to questions. There are no abnormalities in the cardiovascular, respiratory or abdominal systems. There is no lymphadenopathy. On neurological examination, he seems to have mild generalised muscle weakness. Reflexes, tone and sensation are all normal. His peak flow and spirometry measures are within normal limits.

🔍 INVESTIGATIONS

		Normal
Haemoglobin	14.8 g/dL	13.0–17.0 g/dL
Mean corpuscular volume (MCV)	86 fL	80–99 fL
White cell count	6.9 × 10⁹/L	4.0–11.0 × 10⁹/L
Platelets	297 × 10⁹/L	150 400 × 10⁹/L
Sodium	119 mmol/L	135–150 mmol/L
Potassium	3.5 mmol/L	3.4–5.0 mmol/L
Urea	3.1 mmol/L	2.5–7.5 mmol/L
Creatinine	63 µmol/L	70–120 µmol/L

His chest radiograph is shown in Figure 52.1.

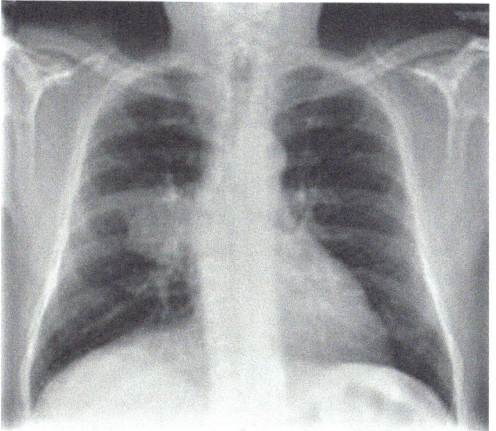

❓ QUESTIONS

- How do you interpret these findings?
- What is the most likely diagnosis?
- What would be the appropriate management?

Figure 52.1 Chest radiograph.

DOI: 10.1201/9781003350934-57

141

ANSWER 52

The blood results show hyponatraemia and the chest radiograph shows a mass overlying the right hilum. This degree of hyponatraemia might be expected to cause some cerebral changes. A lower level might be associated with seizures. Above 120–125 mmol/L, the effects are likely to be non-specific tiredness.

Possible causes for the hyponatraemia in this man are:

- Inappropriate arginine vasopressin (AVP, antidiuretic hormone) secretion in association with the respiratory disorders of lung carcinoma or, occasionally, with pneumonia or tuberculosis; or
- Addison's disease (adrenocortical failure), which would be expected to produce a high potassium level and postural hypotension. Addison's disease might be linked with respiratory problems through adrenal involvement by metastases or tuberculosis.

Other causes, such as diuretic treatment; inappropriate AVP from drug therapy (e.g., carbamazepine, phenothiazines, amitriptyline); cerebrovascular events; salt-losing nephropathies or overhydration from intravenous fluids or over drinking are not likely from the story given here. He has been treated with antidepressants, but not for the last 18 months. In view of the chest radiograph, the most likely diagnosis is inappropriate AVP secretion with a small-cell undifferentiated carcinoma of the lung. This can be confirmed by measurement of serum and urine osmolarities to show serum dilution while the urine is concentrated. Levels of AVP can be measured.

In this case, the osmolarities confirmed the syndrome of inappropriate antidiuretic hormone secretion (SIADH) and bronchial biopsies at fibre-optic bronchoscopy showed a small-cell undifferentiated carcinoma. Extension to the carina and computed tomography (CT) appearances showed it was not resectable. Fluid restriction to 750 mL daily produced an increase in serum sodium to 128 mmol/L with improvement in confusion and weakness. Correction of fluid should be performed carefully to avoid the onset of central pontine demyelination. If this fails to produce adequate results, demeclocycline can be used. This derivative of tetracycline antibiotics interferes with the action of ADH in the renal tubules. Vasopressin antagonists such as tolvaptan are also effective at raising serum sodium, but they are expensive and can cause over-rapid correction.

Chemotherapy was started for the lung tumour. Such treatment often produces a response in terms of shrinkage of the tumour, improved quality of life and increased survival. It may also help the ectopic hormone secretion. Unfortunately, cure is still infrequent. Small-cell undifferentiated carcinomas of the lung are fast-growing tumours, usually unresectable at presentation.

 KEY POINTS

- Change of character may have a metabolic explanation.
- The commonest cause of hyponatraemia is diuretic therapy.
- Measurement of serum and urine osmolarities can help to determine the cause of hyponatraemia.

Section 6
HAEMATOLOGY

CASE 53: PERSONALITY CHANGE

History

A 62-year-old woman is encouraged to consult her general practitioner (GP) because her husband thinks she has become rather confused and irritable over the past 3–4 weeks. She admits to feeling rather annoyed and has found it difficult to remember lists on occasions. There is no relevant medical history.

On systems review, she complains of some non-specific back pain. This has been present for 2 months and is maximal in the low thoracic area. She does not recall any trauma at the start of the problem, and the pain is gradually increasing in severity. It is partially relieved by paracetamol and ibuprofen that she buys in the local pharmacy. She has noticed some abdominal discomfort and constipation, which she has related to the medication for the back pain. She takes no other medicines and does not drink or smoke.

Examination

She looks a little pale. There is no abdominal tenderness. Bowel sounds are normal. She has tenderness locally over the lower thoracic spine.

INVESTIGATIONS

		Normal
Haemoglobin	9.9 g/dL	11.7–15.7 g/dL
White cell count	3.2 × 10⁹/L	3.5–11.0 × 10⁹/L
Platelets	112 × 10⁹/L	150–440 × 10⁹/L
Sodium	140 mmol/L	135–145 mmol/l
Erythrocyte sedimentation rate (ESR)	96 mm/hr	<10 mm/hr
Potassium	3.8 mmol/L	3.5–5.0 mmol/L
Urea	7.5 mmol/L	2.5–6.7 mmol/L
Creatinine	131 µmol/L	70–120 µmol/L
Random glucose	5.1 mmol/L	4.0–6.0 mmol/L

QUESTIONS

- What is the most likely diagnosis?
- What other investigations would you perform?
- What further imaging would you need?

DOI: 10.1201/9781003350934-59

ANSWER 53

There are a number of clues here that there is a significant problem. She presents with a combination of character change, back pain, abdominal pain and constipation. Abdominal pain and constipation might be related to opiate analgesic therapy but not to paracetamol and ibuprofen. The abnormal findings of low values for haemoglobin, white cells and platelets and mildly abnormal renal function are found in the investigations.

The haematological investigations suggest that there is a bone marrow problem, which is likely to be related to the bony tenderness in the thoracic spine. The character change and the abdominal symptoms, with the finding of a possible bony problem, raise the possibility of hypercalcaemia, which would explain all these findings.

The clinical manifestations of hypercalcaemia include confusion, reduced concentration, fatigue, muscle weakness, abdominal pain, nausea, constipation, polydipsia, polyuria, dehydration, nephrolithiasis, hypertension, short QT on electrocardiogram (ECG) and bone changes (osteitis fibrosa cystica, brown tumours).

Ninety percent of cases of hypercalcaemia are related to primary hyperparathyroidism or malignancy, with multiple myeloma as a common malignancy.

> **! OTHER CAUSES ARE:**
>
> - Sarcoidosis
> - Ectopic hormone production in squamous cell lung cancer
> - Tertiary hyperparathyroidism (in renal failure)
> - Thyrotoxicosis
> - Vitamin D intoxication
> - Medications such as lithium, thiazide diuretics (mild hypercalcaemia), calcium-containing antacids
> - Milk-alkali syndrome
> - Adrenal insufficiency
> - Excess growth hormones such as in acromegaly
> - Bone diseases such as Paget's disease
> - Tuberculosis
> - Congenital familial hypocalciuric hypercalcaemia

The investigations indicating bone marrow depression here and the bone pain suggest that malignancy is the likely cause. The high ESR could be compatible with any disseminated malignancy but is characteristic of multiple myeloma.

The important first investigations here are to confirm the hypercalcaemia and to investigate the back pain. When interpreting serum calcium, the serum albumin should be measured and the calcium level corrected for abnormalities in albumin. Also, the serum phosphate may help, being usually low in hyperparathyroidism and high in malignancy. In the presence of hypercalcaemia, the serum parathyroid hormone (PTH) level will be below normal unless there is hyperparathyroidism. Whole-body magnetic resonance imaging (WB-MRI) is recommended in the 2016 NICE guidelines as first-line imaging for all patients with suspected multiple myeloma. It is an effective diagnostic tool to identify any bone marrow involvement, bony lesions and monitoring disease progression. Whole-body low-dose computed tomography (CT) should be considered if WB-MRI is unsuitable for patients and skeletal survey only to be recommended as first-line

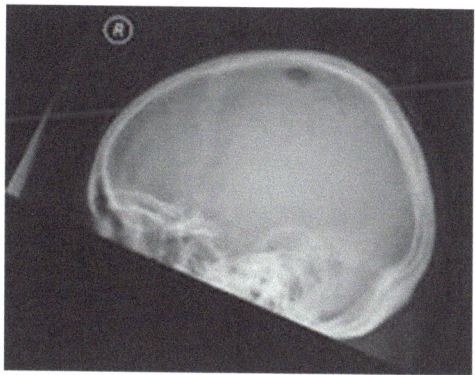

Figure 53.1 Skull radiograph.

imaging if the patient is unsuitable for whole body **MRI** or **CT** imaging. Further investigations to be assessed such as peripheral blood film showing Rouleaux formation in multiple myeloma.

In this case, the serum calcium and phosphate were both raised and the radiographs of the thoracic spine and skull (see Figure 53.1) showed lytic bone lesions typical of multiple myeloma. Plain radiographs are preferred to a radio-isotope bone scan which may not show hot spots from radioisotope accumulation in osteoblasts typical of other malignant bone involvement.

The diagnosis was confirmed with protein electrophoresis, which showed a monoclonal band in the gamma region and by bone marrow biopsy showing an accumulation of abnormal plasma cells. For newly diagnosed multiple myeloma patients who have not had MRI/CT whole body imaging, positron emission tomography (PET)-CT is recommended. Myeloma occurs in about 1–4/100,000 adults per year and is treated by steroids, chemotherapy and stem cell transplants. Remissions are common but cure is unusual.

 KEY POINTS

- Hypercalcaemia symptoms are traditionally stones, bones, abdominal groans and psychic moans, but symptoms may be non-specific.
- Back pain requires investigation when associated with other features such as neurological symptoms or investigations suggesting malignancy or infection.

CASE 54: EASY BRUISING

History

A 68-year-old woman presents to her general practitioner (GP) complaining of spontaneous bruising mainly on her legs. The bruising has been noticeable over the past 3 weeks. She cannot remember any episodes of trauma. She has suffered a major nosebleed. She feels very tired and has noticed shortness of breath on exertion. There is no significant past medical history. There is no family history of a bleeding disorder. She is a non-smoker and drinks a small amount of alcohol socially.

Examination

On examination, there are multiple areas of purpura on her legs and to a lesser extent on her abdomen and arms. The purpuric lesions vary in colour from black–purple to yellow. She is pale with conjunctival pallor. There are two bullae in the mouth and there is spontaneous bleeding from the gums. There are multiple small retinal haemorrhages on fundoscopy. Blood pressure is 118/72 mmHg. Examination of the cardiovascular, respiratory and abdominal systems is unremarkable.

INVESTIGATIONS

		Normal
Haemoglobin	5.8 g/dL	11.7–15.7 g/dL
Mean corpuscular volume (MCV)	83 fL	80–99 fL
White cell count	14.1 × 10⁹/L	3.5–11.0 × 10⁹/L
Platelets	9 × 10⁹/L	150–440 × 10⁹/L
Sodium	139 mmol/L	135–145 mmol/L
Potassium	4.8 mmol/L	3.5–5.0 mmol/L
Urea	4.4 mmol/L	2.5–6.7 mmol/L
Creatinine	85 µmol/L	70–120 µmol/L
Glucose	4.3 mmol/L	4.0–6.0 mmol/L

Clotting screen: normal

QUESTIONS

- What is the differential diagnosis?
- How would you further investigate this patient?
- How would you manage this patient?

ANSWER 54

The combination of anaemia, neutropenia and thrombocytopenia is termed pancytopenia. Causes of severe pancytopenia include aplastic anaemia, vitamin B_{12} or folate deficiency, haematological malignancy such as myelodysplasia or leukaemia and tuberculosis.

This woman has spontaneous bruising due to acute myeloid leukaemia (AML). She has profound thrombocytopenia with a platelet count of 9×10^9/L. An increased tendency to bleed or bruise can be due to platelet, coagulation or blood vessel abnormalities. Platelet/vessel wall defects cause spontaneous purpura in the skin and mucous membranes or immediately after trauma. A lack of a history of trauma and frequent severe bruising raises the possibility of a bleeding diathesis. Disorders of platelet function usually cause immediate bleeding after a procedure, whereas coagulation defects cause haematomas and haemarthroses, usually with a time delay after trauma. The onset of bleeding in later life suggests an acquired condition rather than a congenital cause. Family history may identify a condition such as haemophilia. The distribution of bruising may also suggest the diagnosis. Thrombocytopenic purpura is most evident over the ankles and pressure areas. Retinal haemorrhages tend to occur if there is a combination of severe thrombocytopenia and anaemia. Senile purpura and steroid-induced bruising occur mainly on the forearms and backs of the hands. Henoch-Schönlein purpura typically occur over the extensor aspects of the limbs and buttocks. It is important to take a dietary and drug history. Scurvy causes bleeding from the gums and around the hair follicles. Anticoagulants, antiplatelet drugs and steroids can all cause bruising too.

Petechiae are small capillary haemorrhages that appear as pinhead size lesions and characteristically develop in crops in areas of increased venous pressure. They suggest a problem with platelet number or function. Purpura are larger in size with variable shape and involve bleeding into subcutaneous tissues. Purpura can be seen in a variety of bleeding disorders, including thrombocytopenia and coagulation cascade disorders. Palpable purpura can be seen in vasculitic processes such as Henoch–Schönlein purpura.

AML is the most common acute leukaemia in adults with a mean age at presentation of 65 years. Patients with AML generally present with symptoms related to complications of pancytopenia, including weakness, breathlessness and easy fatigability, infections of variable severity and/or haemorrhagic findings such as gingival bleeding, ecchymoses, epistaxis, or menorrhagia. Most patients will have blasts on the peripheral blood smear and the diagnosis is confirmed by the results of a bone marrow examination.

This patient should be immediately referred to a haematology unit. Platelet transfusion is usually given if there is significant bleeding, or the platelet count is less than 15×10^9/L to prevent a major spontaneous bleed. Initial investigations are examination of the peripheral blood smear and performing a bone marrow aspirate and/or biopsy to confirm the diagnosis and subtype of AML.

 KEY POINTS

- A careful history and examination can help in the diagnosis of easy bruising. The patient should be asked about associated trauma, location and severity of bruising, bleeding history with previous procedures, nutrition, medication use and family history.
- The differential diagnosis of pancytopenia with peripheral blasts includes AML, myelodysplasia, a blast crisis from a chronic myeloid leukaemia, a mixed phenotype acute leukaemia, folate or B_{12} deficiency and miliary tuberculosis.

CASE 55: TIREDNESS, BREATHLESSNESS AND HEADACHES

History

A 63-year-old woman goes to her general practitioner (GP) complaining of extreme tiredness. She has been increasingly fatigued over the past year, but in recent weeks, she has become breathless on exertion and light-headed and complained of headaches. Her feet have become numb, and she has started to become unsteady on her feet. She has had no significant previous medical illnesses. She is a retired teacher and lives alone. Until the past 2 years, she was active, walking 3 or 4 miles a day. She is a non-smoker and drinks about 15 units of alcohol per week. She is taking no regular medication. Her mother and one of her two sisters have thyroid problems.

Examination

Her conjunctivae are pale and sclerae are yellow. Her temperature is 37.8°C. Her pulse rate is 96/min and regular, and blood pressure is 142/72 mmHg. Examination of her cardiovascular, respiratory and abdominal systems is normal. She has a symmetrical distal weakness affecting her arms and legs. Knee and ankle jerks are absent and she has extensor plantar responses. She has sensory loss in a glove-and-stocking distribution with a particularly severe loss of joint position sense.

🔍 INVESTIGATIONS

		Normal
Haemoglobin	4.2 g/dL	11.7–15.7 g/dL
Mean corpuscular volume (MCV)	112 fl	80–99 fL
White cell count	3.3 × 10⁹/L	3.5–11.0 × 10⁹/L
Platelets	102 × 10⁹/L	150–440 × 10⁹/L
Sodium	136 mmol/L	135–145 mmol/L
Potassium	4.4 mmol/L	3.5–5.0 mmol/L
Urea	5.2 mmol/L	2.5–6.7 mmol/L
Creatinine	92 µmol/L	70–120 µmol/L
Glucose	4.4 mmol/L	4.0–6.0 mmol/L
Bilirubin	45 mmol/L	3–17 mmol/L
Alanine transaminase	33 IU/L	5–35 IU/L
Alkaline phosphatase	263 IU/L	30–300 IU/L

? QUESTIONS

- What is the diagnosis?
- How would you investigate this patient?
- How would you manage this patient?

ANSWER 55

This patient has a severe macrocytic anaemia and neurological signs due to vitamin B_{12} deficiency. The alternative diagnoses include hypothyroidism or folate deficiency. There is a family history of thyroid disease; however, the anaemia is too severe for hypothyroidism. Hypothyroidism or folate deficiency would not explain the neurological signs.

Anaemia results in reduced tissue oxygenation. Symptoms include headache, fatigue, breathlessness and dizziness. There is often pallor of the mucous membranes. Profound vitamin B_{12} deficiency causes a peripheral neuropathy and subacute degeneration of the posterior columns and pyramidal tracts in the spinal cord, causing a sensory loss and increased difficulty walking. The peripheral neuropathy and pyramidal tract involvement produce the combination of absent ankle jerks and upgoing plantars. In its most extreme form, it can lead to paraplegia, optic atrophy and dementia.

Vitamin B_{12} is synthesised by micro-organisms and is obtained by ingesting animal or vegetable products contaminated by bacteria. After ingestion, it is bound by intrinsic factor, synthesised by gastric parietal cells, and this complex is then absorbed in the terminal ileum. Vitamin B_{12} deficiency is most commonly of a gastric cause (pernicious anaemia due to an autoimmune atrophic gastritis; total gastrectomy), bacterial overgrowth in the small intestine destroying intrinsic factor or a malabsorption from the terminal ileum (surgical resection; Crohn's disease).

Pernicious anaemia is the most likely cause of this patient's vitamin B_{12} deficiency. Pernicious anaemia is an autoimmune disease with the production of antibodies that inhibit intrinsic factor binding to vitamin B_{12} in the stomach. Vitamin B_{12} cannot be absorbed in the terminal ileum unless it is bound to the intrinsic factor. In pernicious anaemia, the MCV can rise to 100–140 fL and oval macrocytes are seen on the blood film. The reticulocyte count is inappropriately low for the degree of anaemia. The white cell count is usually moderately reduced. There is often a mild rise in serum bilirubin giving the patient a 'lemon-yellow' complexion.

A full dietary history should be taken. Vegans who omit all animal products from their diet often have subclinical vitamin B_{12} deficiency. Serum vitamin B_{12} and folate levels should be measured and anti-intrinsic factor antibodies and anti-gastric parietal cells antibodies should be assayed. Intrinsic factor antibodies are virtually specific for pernicious anaemia but are only present in about 50% of cases. Parietal cell antibody is present in 85–90% of patients with pernicious anaemia but can also occur in patients with other causes of atrophic gastritis. A radioactive B_{12} absorption test (Schilling test) distinguishes gastric from intestinal causes of deficiency. However, the Schilling test is no longer routinely performed.

Rapid correction of vitamin B_{12} is essential using intramuscular hydroxycobalamin (3 times per week, for 2 weeks followed by 3 monthly B_{12} injections) to prevent cardiac failure and further neurological damage. Folic acid supplement may also be recommended.

> **! DIFFERENTIAL DIAGNOSES OF MACROCYTIC ANAEMIA**
>
> - Folate deficiency
> - Excessive alcohol consumption
> - Hypothyroidism
> - Certain drugs (e.g., azathioprine, methotrexate)
> - Primary acquired sideroblastic anaemia and myelodysplastic syndromes

KEY POINTS

- Vitamin B_{12} deficiency may occur in strict vegetarians who eat no dairy products.
- Typical neurological signs are position and vibration sense impairment in the legs, absent reflexes and extensor plantars.
- Overenthusiastic blood transfusion should be avoided since it can provoke cardiac failure in vitamin B_{12} deficiency.

CASE 56: SWELLING IN THE NECK

History

A 38-year-old man presents to his general practitioner (GP) complaining of a painless lump on the right side of his neck. This has been present for about 2 months and seems to be enlarging. He has had no recent throat infections. He has been feeling generally unwell and has lost about 5 kg in weight. The patient has also developed drenching night sweats. Simultaneously, he has noticed severe generalised itching. He has had no significant past medical history. He is an accountant and is married with three children. He neither smokes nor drinks alcohol and is not taking any regular medication.

Examination

His temperature is 37.8°C. There is a smooth, firm 3 × 4 cm palpable mass in the right supra-clavicular fossae. There are also lymph nodes 1–2 cm in diameter, palpable in both axillae and inguinal areas. His oropharynx appears normal. There are multiple excoriations of his skin. His pulse rate is 100/min and regular, and blood pressure is 112/66 mmHg. Examination of his cardiovascular and respiratory systems is normal. On abdominal examination, there is a mass palpable 3 cm below the left costal margin. The mass is dull to percussion, and it is impossible to palpate its upper edge. Neurological examination is normal.

🔍 INVESTIGATIONS

		Normal
Haemoglobin	11.6 g/dL	13.3–17.7 g/dL
Mean corpuscular volume (MCV)	87 fL	80–99 fL
White cell count	12.2 × 10⁹/L	3.9–10.6 × 10⁹/L
Platelcts	321 × 10⁹/L	150–440 × 10⁹/L
Erythrocyte sedimentation rate	74 mm/h	<10 mm/h
Sodium	138 mmol/L	135–145 mmol/L
Potassium	4.2 mmol/L	3.5–5.0 mmol/L
Urea	5.2 mmol/L	2.5–6.7 mmol/L
Creatinine	114 µmol/L	70–120 µmol/L
Calcium	2.44 mmol/L	2.12–2.65 mmol/L
Phosphate	1.1 mmol/L	0.8–1.45 mmol/L
Total protein	65 g/L	60–80 g/L
Albumin	41 g/L	35–50 g/L
Bilirubin	16 mmol/L	3–17 mmol/L
Alanine transaminase	22 IU/L	5–35 IU/L
Alkaline phosphatase	228 IU/L	30–300 IU/L

Urinalysis: no protein; no blood

❓ QUESTIONS

- What is the likely diagnosis?
- How would you investigate this patient?
- How would you manage this patient?

ANSWER 56

Transient small nodes in the neck or groin are common benign findings. However, a 3×4 cm mass of nodes for 2 months is undoubtedly abnormal. Persistent lymphadenopathy and constitutional symptoms suggest a likely diagnosis of lymphoma or chronic leukaemia. Sarcoidosis and tuberculosis are possible but less likely diagnoses. Lymph nodes are normally barely palpable, if at all. The character of enlarged lymph nodes is very important. In acute infections, the nodes are tender and the overlying skin may be red. Carcinomatous nodes are usually very hard, fixed and irregular. The nodes of chronic leukaemias and lymphomas are non-tender, firm and rubbery. The distribution of enlarged lymph nodes may be diagnostic. Repeated minor trauma and infection may cause enlargement of the locally draining lymph nodes. Enlargement of the left supraclavicular nodes may be due to metastatic spread from bronchial and nasopharyngeal carcinomas or from gastric carcinomas (Virchow's node). However, when there is generalised lymphadenopathy with or without splenomegaly, a systemic illness is most likely. The typical systemic symptoms of lymphoma are malaise, fever, night sweats, pruritus, weight loss, anorexia and fatigue. Fever indicates extensive disease and may be associated with night sweats. Severe skin itching is a feature of some cases of lymphoma and other myeloproliferative illnesses.

The incidence of lymphoma is greatly increased in patients who are immunosuppressed, such as organ transplant recipients and patients with human immunodeficiency virus (HIV) infection.

!   MAJOR DIFFERENTIAL DIAGNOSIS OF GENERALISED LYMPHADENOPATHY

- **Infections:** Infectious mononucleosis or 'glandular fever' (caused by Epstein-Barr virus infection), toxoplasmosis, cytomegalovirus infection, acute HIV infection, tuberculosis, brucellosis and syphilis.
- **Inflammatory conditions:** Systemic lupus erythematosus, rheumatoid arthritis and sarcoidosis.
- **Malignancy:** Lymphomas or chronic lymphocytic leukaemia.

The most likely clinical diagnosis in this man is lymphoma. The patient should be referred to a local haemato-oncology unit. He should have a lymph node biopsy to reach a histological diagnosis and a computed tomography (CT) scan of the thorax, abdomen and bone marrow to stage the disease. CT scanning is a non-invasive and effective method of imaging retroperitoneal, iliac and mesenteric nodes. Positron emission tomography (PET) combined with CT increases the sensitivity for detecting disease (Figure 56.1) and is useful for assessing response to treatment.

The patient will require treatment with chemotherapy, and perhaps radiotherapy in addition. Radiotherapy alone is reserved for patients with limited disease, but this patient has widespread disease. He should be given allopurinol prior to starting chemotherapy to prevent massive release of uric acid as a consequence of tumour lysis, which can cause acute renal failure.

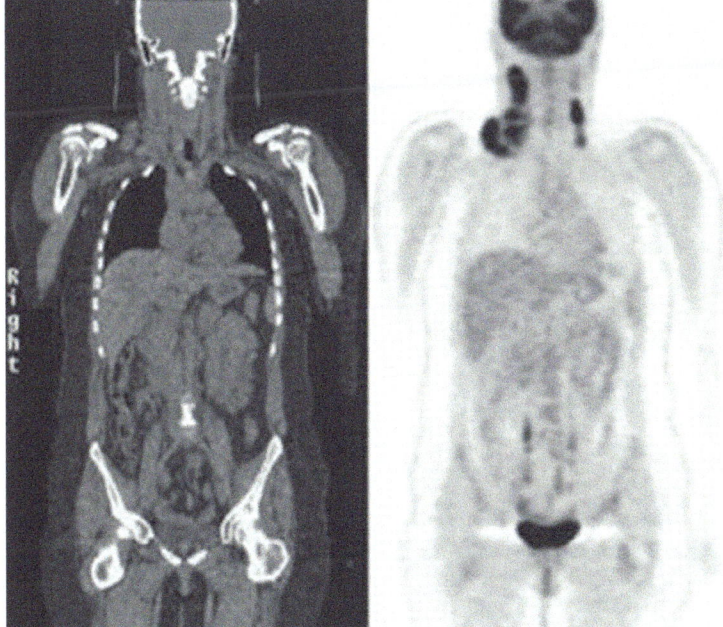

Figure 56.1 CT-PET image showing increased activity in enlarged lymph nodes, particularly in the right side of the neck.

 KEY POINTS

- The character and distribution of abnormal lymph nodes is helpful in reaching a diagnosis.
- Lymphadenopathy affecting two or more separate groups of nodes suggests lymphoma or a systemic infection.
- CT-PET scanning allows accurate staging of disease and assessment of maintenance of remission in response to treatment.

CASE 57: PAIN IN THE CHEST AND SHORTNESS OF BREATH

History

A 17-year-old African-Caribbean boy presents to the emergency department complaining of severe chest pain and shortness of breath. He has had a sore throat for a few days and started developing pain in his back and arms, which has increased in severity. Six hours prior to admission, he suddenly developed right-sided chest pain, which is worse on inspiration and associated with marked breathlessness. He has had previous episodes of pains affecting his fingers and back, for which he has taken codeine and ibuprofen. He was born in London and lives with his parents and younger sister. There is no family history of note.

Examination

He is unwell, febrile (37.8°C) and cyanosed. His conjunctivae are pale. Pulse rate is 112/min and regular, and blood pressure is 136/85 mmHg. His jugular venous pressure is not raised, and heart sounds are normal. His respiratory rate is 28/min, and a right pleural rub is audible. Abdominal and neurological examination is normal. There are no rashes on the skin and no joint abnormalities.

🔍 INVESTIGATIONS

		Normal
Haemoglobin	7.6 g/dL	13.3–17.7 g/dL
Mean corpuscular volume (MCV)	86 fL	80–99 fL
White cell count	16×10^9/L	$3.9–10.6 \times 10^9$/L
Platelets	182×10^9/L	$150–440 \times 10^9$/L
Sodium	139 mmol/L	135–145 mmol/L
Potassium	4.4 mmol/L	3.5–5.0 mmol/L
Urea	6.2 mmol/L	2.5–6.7 mmol/L
Creatinine	94 µmol/L	70–120 µmol/L
Bicarbonate	21 mmol/L	24–30 mmol/L
Arterial blood gases on air:		
pH	7.33	7.38–7.44
pCO$_2$	2.6 kPa	4.7–6.0 kPa
pO$_2$	7.2 kPa	12.0–14.5 kPa

Electrocardiogram (ECG): sinus tachycardia
Chest radiograph: normal

❓ QUESTIONS

- What is the likely diagnosis?
- How would you investigate this patient?
- How would you manage this patient?

ANSWER 57

This boy has sickle cell disease and presents with his first serious bony/chest crisis. Sickle cell disease occurs mainly in African black populations and sporadically in the Mediterranean and Middle East. Haemoglobin S differs from haemoglobin A by the substitution of valine for glutamic acid at position 6 in the b-chain. Sickled cells have increased mechanical fragility and a shortened survival, leading to haemolytic anaemia, and can block small vessels, leading to tissue infarction. Sickle cell disease has a variable clinical course due to a combination of reasons, including the haemoglobin F (HbF) level and socioeconomic factors. It usually presents in early childhood with anaemia and jaundice due to chronic haemolytic anaemia or painful hands and feet with inflammation of the fingers due to dactylitis. This patient is having a pulmonary crisis characterised by pleuritic chest pain, shortness of breath and hypoxia. It is usually precipitated by dehydration or infection (in this case, a sore throat). The principal differential diagnoses of a patient presenting with pleuritic pain and breathlessness are pneumonia, pneumothorax and pulmonary emboli.

! MAJOR POTENTIAL COMPLICATIONS OF SICKLE CELL DISEASE

- **Thrombotic:** Causes generalised or localised bony pains, abdominal crises, chest crises, neurological signs or priapism.
- **Aplastic crises:** Triggered by parvovirus infection.
- **Haemolytic anaemia**.
- **Sequestration crises** in children with rapid enlargement of the liver and spleen, usually in young children.
- **Aseptic necrosis:** Often of the humeral or femoral heads.
- **Renal failure** due to renal medullary infarction or glomerular disease.
- **Hyposplenism** due to autoinfarction in childhood.

The definitive investigation is haemoglobin electrophoresis, which will demonstrate HbS, absent HbA and a variable HbF level. Partial exchange transfusion may be needed to reduce the level of his sickle cells to less than 30%.

This patient should be admitted for rest, intravenous fluids, oxygen and adequate analgesia. He has a low arterial pO_2 and appears cyanosed. Cyanosis is more difficult to detect in the presence of anaemia. Infection should be treated with antibiotics. A blood film will show sickled erythrocytes and elevated reticulocyte count. He should be followed up by an expert sickle team since this has been shown to reduce admissions and improve quality of care. He may benefit from long-term hydroxyurea, which raises the HbF level and reduces the number of crises. NICE guidelines recommended patients with sickle cell to receive pneumococcal vaccine every 5 years.

🔑 KEY POINTS

- In African-Caribbean patients, sickle cell disease should be thought of as a cause of chest or abdominal pain.
- Patients with sickle cell disease should be looked after in specialised haematology units with psychological support available.
- Severe thrombotic complications should be treated with partial exchange transfusion.

Section 7
RESPIRATORY

CASE 58: CHRONIC COUGH

History

A 19-year-old boy has a history of repeated chest infections. He had problems with a cough and sputum production in the first 2 years of life and was labelled as bronchitic. Over the next 14 years, he was often 'chesty' and had spent 4 to 5 weeks a year away from school. Over the past 2 years, he has developed more problems and was admitted to hospital on three occasions with cough and purulent sputum. On the first two occasions, *Haemophilus influenzae* was grown on culture of the sputum, and on the last occasion 2 months ago, *Pseudomonas aeruginosa* was isolated from the sputum at the time of admission to hospital. He is still coughing up sputum. Although he has largely recovered from the infection, his mother is worried and asked for a further sputum sample to be sent off. The report has come back from the microbiology laboratory showing that there is a scanty growth of *Pseudomonas* on culture of the sputum.

There is no family history of any chest disease. Routine questioning shows that his appetite is reasonable, micturition is normal and his bowels tend to be irregular.

Examination

On examination he is thin, weighing 48 kg, and is 1.6 m (5 ft 6 in) tall.

- The only finding in the chest is of a few inspiratory crackles over the upper zones of both lungs. Cardiovascular and abdominal examination is normal.

 INVESTIGATIONS

The chest radiograph is shown in Figure 58.1.

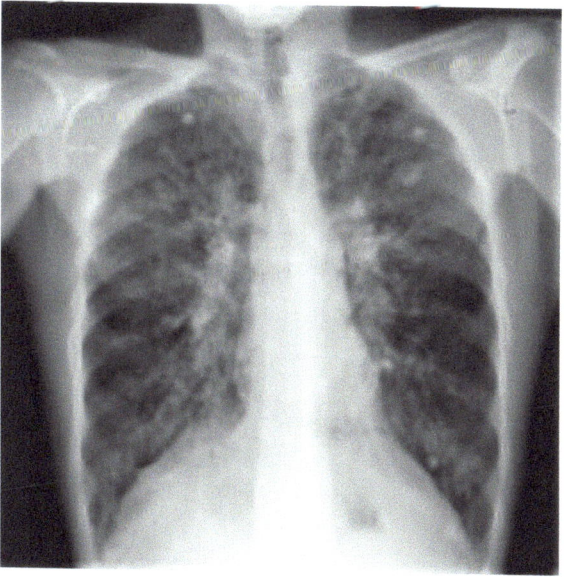

Figure 58.1 Chest radiograph.

? **QUESTIONS**

- What does the radiograph show?
- What is the most likely diagnosis?
- What investigations should be performed?

ANSWER 58

The chest radiograph shows abnormal shadowing throughout both lungs, more marked in the upper lobes, with some ring shadows and tubular shadows representing thickened bronchial walls. These findings would be compatible with a diagnosis of bronchiectasis. The pulmonary arteries are prominent, suggesting a degree of pulmonary hypertension. The distribution is typical of that found in cystic fibrosis, where the changes are most evident in the upper lobes. Most other forms of bronchiectasis are more likely to occur in the lower lobes, where drainage by gravity is less effective. Sputum analysis aids diagnosis; however, high-resolution chest computed tomography (CT) is the confirmatory test to diagnose bronchiectasis and define its extent and distribution. In young children with cystic fibrosis, the predominant organisms detected in the sputum are *Haemophilus influenzae* and *Staphylococcus aureus*. In older children and adults, *Pseudomonas aeruginosa* is the most common pathogen, present in about 25% of patients. Once present in the lungs, it is difficult to remove completely. Chronic infection of *Pseudomonas aeruginosa* is associated with accelerated decline of lung function and a poorer prognosis.

Cystic fibrosis should always be considered when there is a history of repeated chest infections in a young person. Although it most often presents before the age of 20, diagnosis may be delayed until in their 20s–40s or later in milder cases. Associated problems occur in the pancreas (malabsorption, diabetes), sinuses and liver. It has become evident that some patients are affected more mildly, especially those with the less-common genetic variants. These milder cases may only be affected by the chest features of cystic fibrosis and have little or no malabsorption from the pancreatic insufficiency.

> **! DIFFERENTIAL DIAGNOSIS OF DIFFUSE BRONCHIECTASIS**
>
> - **Agammaglobulinaemia**
> - **Immotile cilia**
> - **Tuberculosis – bronchiectasis of the upper lobes**
> - **Allergic bronchopulmonary aspergillosis associated with asthma**
>
> Respiratory function should be measured to see the degree of functional impairment.

In the UK, most cases of cystic fibrosis are picked up at birth using the newborn screening heel-prick test, which looks for raised immunoreactive trypsin levels within the blood. The most conclusive test for diagnosis in both children and adults is the sweat test where electrolytes in the sweat are measured. In cystic fibrosis, there is an abnormally high concentration of sodium and chloride. Genetic testing can also be used to diagnose cystic fibrosis. In the rare case of people with symptoms who have normal sweat or gene test results, diagnosis can be made by clinical manifestations alone.

Cystic fibrosis has an autosomal recessive inheritance with the commonest genetic abnormality ΔF508 found in 70% of cases. The CFTR gene is responsible for the protein controlling chloride transport across the cell membrane. In cystic fibrosis, mutations in the CFTR gene can lead to a cascade of problems affecting primarily the lungs and the gastrointestinal system. Since the identification of the genetic abnormality, trials of gene-replacement therapy have begun, with the potential for clinical trials to begin in the next several years.

First-line management involves chest physiotherapy accompanied by a short-acting bronchodilator and inhaled mucolytics to mobilise secretions from the airway walls into the lumen where they can be coughed out. Other management considerations include oral or inhaled antibiotics and anti-inflammatory agents in chronic infection states, as well as non-invasive ventilation during flare ups. For patients who are homozygous for the ΔF508 mutation, lumacaftor/ivacaftor (Orkambi) can be tried, which works by increasing the number of CFTR proteins transported to the cell surface. In later stages, when all alternative therapies have been exhausted, bilateral lung transplantation can be considered.

 KEY POINTS

- Milder forms of cystic fibrosis may present in adolescence and adulthood.
- Milder forms are often related to less-common genetic abnormalities.
- A high-resolution CT scan is the best way to detect bronchiectasis and to define its extent.
- Management involves chest physiotherapy, short-acting bronchodilators and mucolytics.

CASE 59: SHORTNESS OF BREATH

History

A 26-year-old teacher has consulted her general practitioner (GP) for her persistent cough. She wants to have a second course of antibiotics because an initial course of amoxicillin made no difference. The cough has troubled her for 3 months, since she moved to a new school. The cough is now disturbing her sleep and making her tired during the day. She teaches games, and the cough is troublesome when going out to the playground and when jogging. She had her appendix removed 3 years ago. She had her tonsils removed as a child and was said to have recurrent episodes of bronchitis between the ages of 3 and 6 years. She has never smoked and takes no medication other than an oral contraceptive. Her parents are alive and well, and she has two brothers, one of whom has hay fever.

Examination

The respiratory rate is 18/min. Her chest is clear, and there are no abnormalities in the nose or pharynx or the cardiovascular, respiratory or nervous systems.

🔍 **INVESTIGATIONS**

Chest radiograph is reported as normal.
Spirometry is carried out at the surgery, and she is asked to record her peak flow rate at home, the best of three readings every morning and every evening for 2 weeks. Spirometry results are as follows:

	Actual	Predicted
FEV$_1$ (L)	3.9	3.6–4.2
FVC (L)	5.0	4.5–5.4
FER (FEV$_1$/FVC) (%)	78	75–80
PEF (L/min)	470	440–540

Abbreviations: FEV$_1$: forced expiratory volume in 1 s; FVC: forced vital capacity; FER: forced expiratory ratio; PEF: peak expiratory flow.

A peak flow recording is shown in Figure 59.1.

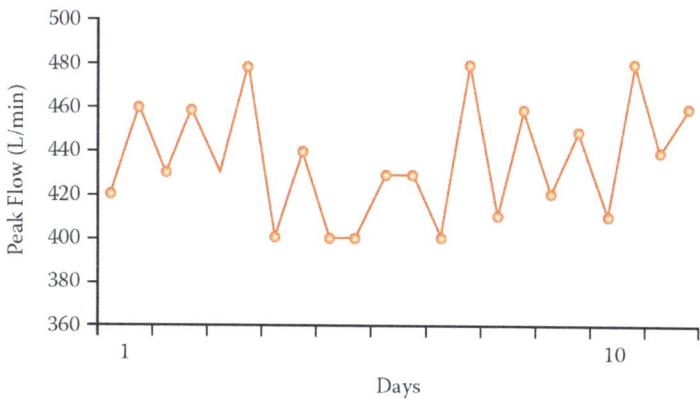

Figure 59.1 Peak flow recording at home over 11 days.

DOI: 10.1201/9781003350934-66

? **QUESTIONS**

- What is your interpretation of these findings?
- What do you think is the likely diagnosis?
- What would be an appropriate treatment?

ANSWER 59

The peak flow pattern shows a degree of diurnal variation. This does not reach the diagnostic criteria for asthma, but it is suspicious. The mean daily variation in peak flow from the recordings is 36 L/min and the mean evening peak flow is 453 L/min, giving a mean diurnal variation of 8%. There is a small diurnal variation in normals, and a variation of >10% is positive for excessive variability, which would support an asthma diagnosis. In this patient, the label of 'bronchitis' as a child was probably asthma. The family history of an atopic condition (hay fever in a brother) and the triggering of the cough by exercise and going out in the cold also suggest bronchial hyperresponsiveness typical of asthma.

Patients with a chronic persistent cough of unexplained cause should have a chest radiograph. When the radiograph is clear, the cough is likely to be produced by one of three main causes in non-smokers. About half of such cases have asthma or will go on to develop asthma over the next few years. A quarter have rhinitis or sinusitis with a postnasal drip. In about 20%, the cough is related to gastro-oesophageal reflux. A small number of cases will be caused by otherwise-unsuspected problems such as foreign bodies, bronchial 'adenoma', sarcoidosis or fibrosing alveolitis. Cough is a common side effect in patients treated with angiotensin-converting enzyme (ACE) inhibitors.

The diagnosis of asthma was confirmed with a bronchodilator reversibility test where reversibility of airflow obstruction to a short-acting bronchodilator was demonstrated. This is defined as an improvement in FEV_1 greater than 12% and greater than 200 ml from baseline. Exercise-induced symptoms may occur in up to 90% of people with asthma. In this patient's exercise test, a 25% drop in FEV_1 was seen after completion of 6 minutes of vigorous exercise. Exercise-induced bronchoconstriction is diagnosed on a percentage fall in FEV_1 of greater than 10% after exercise. Challenge tests such as a bronchoprovocation test may be considered to support the diagnosis if spirometry and PEF does not show reversibility and variability. This includes the use of inhaled methacholine or histamine, and a fall in FEV_1 greater than 20%. Another established diagnostic test is by measuring the fractional exhaled nitric oxide (FeNO) level produced by inducible nitric oxide synthase (iNOS). Nitric oxide (NO) levels tend to rise with inflammatory cells such as eosinophils, which play a significant role in the pathophysiology of asthma. Therefore, the levels of NO typically correlate with the levels of airway inflammation. In adults, a FeNO level of 40 ppb or more is considered positive for asthma.

After the exercise test and a diagnosis of severely uncontrolled asthma, an inhaled steroid was given, and the cough settled after 1 week. The inhaled steroid was discontinued after 4 weeks and replaced by a short-acting beta-agonist (SABA) to use before exercise. However, the cough recurred with more evident wheeze and shortness of breath, and treatment was changed back to an inhaled steroid with a SABA as needed. If control was not established, the next step would be to check inhaler technique and treatment adherence and to consider adding a leukotriene receptor antagonist (LTRA) e.g., montelukast. Long-acting beta-agonist (LABA) can be given if symptoms remain uncontrolled after using LTRA. In some cases, the persistent dry cough associated with asthma may require more vigorous treatment than this. Inhaled steroids for a month or more or even a 2-week course of oral steroids may be needed to relieve the cough. The successful management of dry cough relies on establishing the correct diagnosis and treating it vigorously.

KEY POINTS

- The three commonest causes of persistent dry cough with a normal chest radiograph are asthma (50%), sinusitis and postnasal drip (25%) and reflux oesophagitis (20%).
- Asthma may present as a cough (cough-variant asthma) with little or no airflow obstruction initially, although this develops later.
- Persistent cough with normal chest examination is unlikely to have a bacterial cause or respond to antibiotic treatment.

CASE 60: FEVER AND SHORTNESS OF BREATH

History

A 62-year-old man presents to the emergency department complaining of shortness of breath. Four days prior, he felt unwell with muscle aches and headache. The next day, he developed rigors, dry cough and shortness of breath. His wife recorded a temperature of 39°C. She called an ambulance when his breathing worsened and he became disoriented. There is no significant past medical history. He is a non-smoker and drinks 20 units of alcohol a week. Ten days prior to admission, he had returned from a coach tour of Spain and Portugal.

Examination

On examination he looks unwell, dehydrated and flushed. His temperature is 39.5°C. He has central cyanosis. His pulse rate is 120/min and blood pressure is 146/72 mmHg. His respiratory rate is 32/min and oxygen saturation is 86% breathing room air. His trachea is central and chest expansion is symmetrical. Percussion is reduced at the bases posteriorly and auscultation reveals bilateral crackles and bronchial breathing in both lower zones posteriorly. His abdomen is diffusely tender, but there is no rigidity or guarding. He is disorientated in time, place and person.

Blood tests, arterial blood gases on air, urinalysis and chest radiograph (Figure 60.1) are shown in the table.

INVESTIGATIONS

		Normal
Haemoglobin	15.3 g/dL	13.3–17.7 g/dL
White cell count	10.3 × 10^9/L	3.9–10.6 × 10^9/L
Neutrophils	8.9 × 10^9/L	1.8–7.7 × 10^9/L
Lymphocytes	0.4 × 10^9/L	0.6–4.8 × 10^9/L
Platelets	143 × 10^9/L	150–440 × 10^9/L
Sodium	124 mmol/L	135–145 mmol/L
Potassium	4.4 mmol/L	3.5–5.0 mmol/L
Urea	14.4 mmol/L	2.5–6.7 mmol
Creatinine	178 µmol/L	70–120 µmol/L
Glucose	7.7 mmol/L	4.0–6.0 mmol/L
Calcium	1.88 mmol/L	2.12–2.65 mmol/L
Phosphate	1.2 mmol/L	0.8–1.45 mmol/L
C-reactive protein (CRP)	256 mg/L	<5 mg/L
Arterial blood gases on air		
pH	7.38	7.38–7.44
pCO_2	2.7 kPa	4.7–6.0 kPa
pO_2	6.3 kPa	12.0–14.5 kPa

Urinalysis: ++ blood; ++ protein

DOI: 10.1201/9781003350934-67

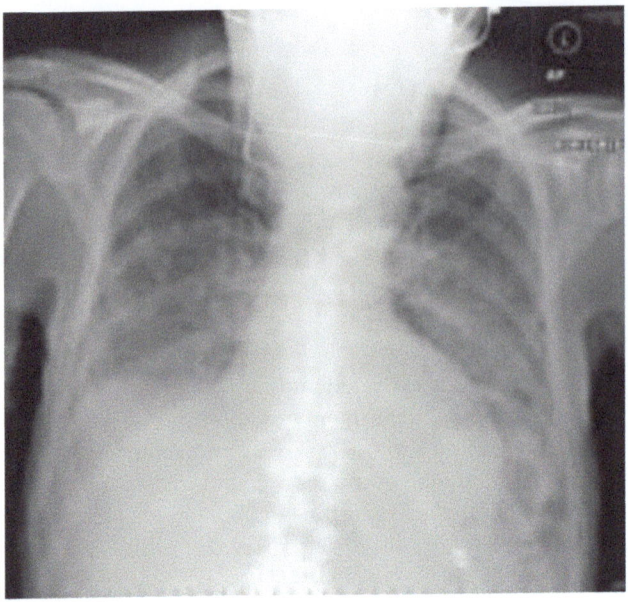

Figure 60.1 Chest radiograph.

? | **QUESTIONS**

- What is the likely diagnosis?
- How would you further investigate this patient?
- How would you manage this patient?

ANSWER 60

This is community acquired pneumonia (CAP) and the most likely organism given the history, symptoms and investigations is *Legionella pneumophila* (Legionnaires' disease).

CAP is most commonly caused by *Streptococcus pneumoniae* or *Haemophilus influenzae*, but atypical pneumonias (pneumonias caused by 'atypical' organisms such as mycoplasma, legionella and chlamydia, which are difficult to detect through standard methods and aren't penicillin sensitive), account for about 5–15% of cases. The 4-day prodromal illness is typical of *Legionella* pneumonia (2–10 days) compared to pneumococcal pneumonia, which tends to present abruptly with fever and shortness of breath. *Legionella* infection presents with malaise, myalgia, headache and fever. Patients may develop diarrhoea and abdominal pain. As the illness progresses, the patient develops a dry cough, chest pain, shortness of breath and acute confusion.

On examination, the patient is usually dehydrated, tachycardic and tachypnoeic, with widespread rhonchi and crackles.

The diffuse infiltrates on chest radiograph suggest atypical pneumonia or viral pneumonia, whereas a lobar pattern tends to occur with streptococcal pneumonia. Hyponatremia occurs in cases of severe pneumonia and is a poor prognostic factor. Confusion and raised urea are markers of severity (used in the CURB65 criteria of severity). The high CRP is consistent with a severe infection. The patient's arterial blood gases showed marked hypoxia with compensatory increased ventilation producing the low $PaCO_2$.

Other potential complications include nephritis, endocarditis and myocarditis.

This patient presumably acquired his infection while on holiday in Spain or Portugal. Legionella outbreaks have been linked to contaminated water tanks and air conditioning units in institutions such as hotels and hospitals.

This man is acutely unwell and should be admitted to a high-dependency unit. He needs a high concentration of inspired oxygen (or ventilatory support if necessary) and intravenous fluids to correct his dehydration. He should be started on intravenous antibiotics promptly, ideally after blood cultures are collected.

Other microbiological tests include urinary antigen testing – this is a rapid, simple test to detect *Legionella* and streptococcal antigens. Sputum cultures should also be collected as well as a respiratory viral throat swab (severe viral pneumonias may have a similar presentation).

Local antibiotic guidelines should be followed for CAP – a typical combination will include a beta-lactam to treat common causes and a macrolide, quinolone or tetracycline to treat the aforementioned 'atypical' causes. Levofloxacin is an antibiotic with good efficacy against *Legionella*.

 KEY POINTS

- *Legionella* is one of the atypical causes of pneumonia.
- It should be suspected if there is a history of water exposure, an outbreak in an institution or if a case of pneumonia fails to respond to antibiotics.
- *Legionella* pneumonia has a 2–10 day prodromal period.
- Hyponatremia and confusion are other clues to the diagnosis.

CASE 61: CHEST PAIN AND SHORTNESS OF BREATH

History

A 29-year-old woman complained of a sudden onset of right-sided chest pain with shortness of breath. It woke her from sleep at 3:00 am. The pain was made worse by a deep breath and by coughing. The breathlessness persisted over 4 hours from its onset to her arrival in the emergency department. She has a slight non-productive cough. There is no relevant previous medical history except asthma controlled by salbutamol and beclomethasone. There is no family history of note. She works as a driving instructor and returned from a 3-week holiday in Australia 3 weeks previously. She had no illnesses while she was away. She has taken an oral contraceptive for the last 4 years.

Examination

She has a temperature of 37.4°C, her respiratory rate is 24/min, the jugular venous pressure is raised 3 cm, blood pressure is 110/64 mmHg and the pulse rate is 128/min. Peak flow rate is 410 L/min. In the respiratory system, expansion is reduced because of pain. Percussion and tactile vocal fremitus are normal and equal. A pleural rub can be heard over the right lower zone posteriorly. There are no other added sounds. Otherwise, the examination is normal.

🔍 **INVESTIGATIONS**

- An electrocardiogram (ECG) is shown in Figure 61.1.
- Figure 61.2 shows her chest radiograph.

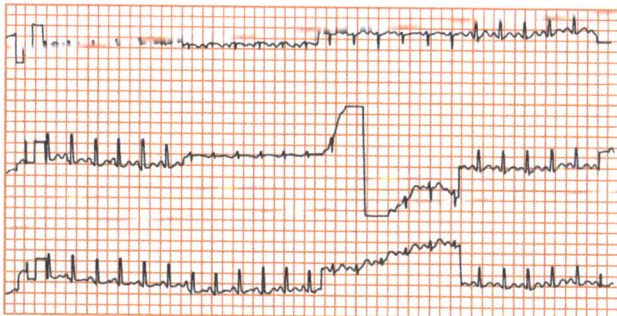

Figure 61.1 Electrocardiogram.

DOI: 10.1201/9781003350934-68

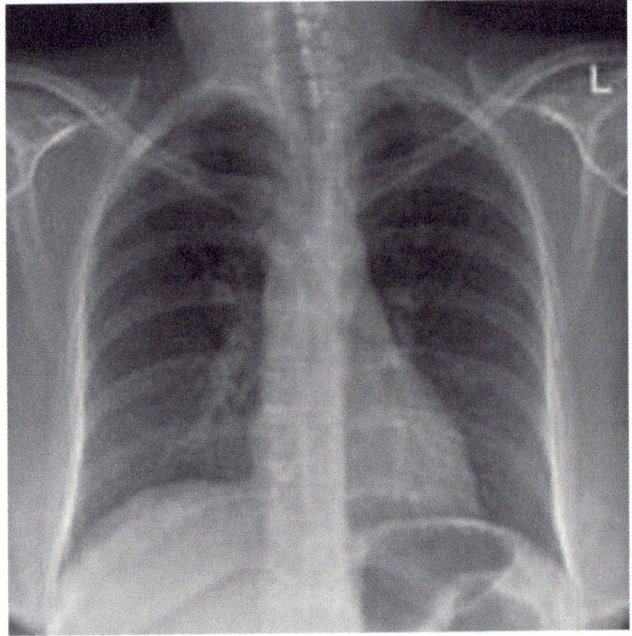

Figure 61.2 Chest radiograph.

? │ **QUESTIONS**

- What is the likely diagnosis?
- How can it be confirmed?
- How should this patient be managed?

ANSWER 61

This woman has had a sudden onset of pleuritic pain, breathlessness and cough. The physical signs of tachypnoea, tachycardia, raised jugular venous pressure and pleural rub would fit with a diagnosis of a pulmonary embolus. The peak flow of 410 L/min indicates that asthma does not explain her breathlessness.

The differential diagnosis would include pneumonia, pneumothorax and pulmonary embolism. The clinical signs do not suggest pneumothorax or pneumonia. Possible predisposing factors for pulmonary embolism are the history of a long aeroplane journey 3 weeks earlier, oral contraception and her work involving sitting for prolonged periods. Other predisposing factors, such as intravenous drug abuse, should be considered. The ECG shows sinus tachycardia. The often-quoted pattern of S-wave in lead I, Q-wave and T inversion in lead III (S1Q3T3) is not common except with massive pulmonary embolus. Other signs, such as transient right ventricular hypertrophy features, P pulmonale and T-wave changes, may also occur. The chest radiograph is normal, ruling out pneumothorax and lobar pneumonia.

A computed tomographic pulmonary angiography (CTPA) is the preferred investigation for definitive confirmation of PE. This will provide direct visualisation of the thrombus. A ventilation–perfusion lung scan could be done to look for a typical mismatch with an area that is ventilated but not perfused. This result would have a high probability for a diagnosis of pulmonary embolism. In cases with a normal chest radiograph and no history of chronic lung disease, equivocal results are less common, and it is not usually necessary to go further than the lung scan. In the presence of chronic lung disease such as chronic obstructive pulmonary disease (COPD) or significant asthma, the ventilation–perfusion lung scan is more likely to be equivocal and further tests are more often used. In this case, a CTPA was carried out (Figure 61.3). This showed a filling defect typical of an embolus in the right lower lobe pulmonary artery.

A search for a source of emboli with a Doppler of the leg veins may help in some cases, and the finding of negative D-dimers in the blood makes intravascular thrombosis and embolism unlikely.

Initial supportive treatment for a haemodynamically unstable patient includes respiratory support. Further immediate management should involve unfractionated heparin initially.

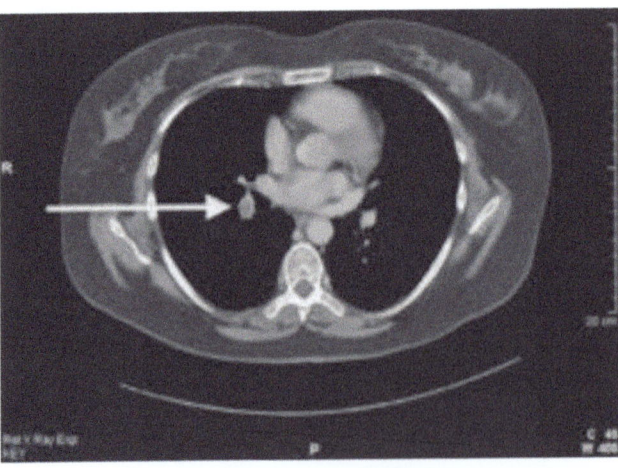

Figure 61.3 Computed tomography pulmonary angiogram.

The anticoagulation can then transfer to a direct oral anticoagulant (DOAC) such as apixaban or subcutaneous low-molecular-weight heparin (LMWH). Alternative modes of contraception should be discussed and advice given on alternating walking or other leg movements with her seated periods at work. Thrombolysis should be considered when there is haemodynamic compromise by a large embolus. Provoked pulmonary embolism (i.e., when risk factors are present) is usually treated with 3 months of anticoagulation, while unprovoked pulmonary embolism (i.e., when none of the risk factors is present) is treated for 6 months. For patients with recurrent pulmonary embolism, an inferior vena cava filter (a special basket-like metal device designed to trap clots) can be inserted through a small incision in a vein in the groin or neck.

 KEY POINTS

- In the presence of a normal chest radiograph and no chronic lung disease, the ventilation–perfusion lung scan has good sensitivity and specificity.
- The chest radiograph and ECG are often unhelpful in the diagnosis of pulmonary embolism.
- CTPA is used when ventilation–perfusion scanning is likely to be unhelpful.

CASE 62: CHEST PAIN AND SHORTNESS OF BREATH

History

A 25-year-old female accountant complains of shortness of breath, cough and chest pain. The chest pain came on suddenly, about 6 hours ago when she was walking to work. It was a sharp pain in the right side of her chest. The pain was made worse by breathing. It settled over the next few hours, but there is still a mild ache in the right side on deep breathing. She felt a little short of breath for the first hour or two after the pain came on, but now only feels this on stairs or walking quickly. She has had a dry cough throughout the 6 hours.

She smokes 15 cigarettes a day and drinks 10 units of alcohol a week. She uses marijuana occasionally. She is not on any medication. Four years ago, something very similar happened; she is not sure but thinks that the pain was on the left side of the chest on that occasion. There is no relevant family history.

Examination

She is not distressed or cyanosed. Her pulse is 88/min and blood pressure is 128/78 mmHg; respiratory rate is 20/min. Heart sounds are normal. In the respiratory system, the trachea and apex beat are not displaced. Expansion seems normal, as is percussion. There is decreased tactile vocal fremitus and the intensity of the breath sounds is reduced over the right side of the chest. There are no added sounds on auscultation.

 INVESTIGATIONS

The chest radiograph is shown in Figure 62.1.

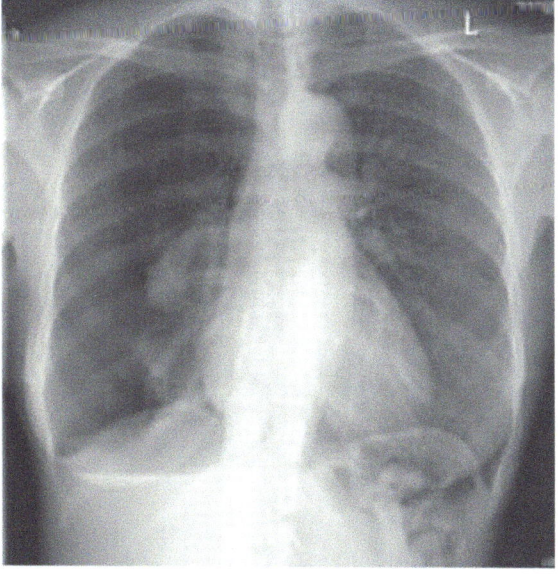

Figure 62.1 Chest radiograph.

? **QUESTIONS**

- What does the radiograph show?
- What should be done now?
- What further advice should be given to this patient?

DOI: 10.1201/9781003350934-69

ANSWER 62

The chest radiograph shows a large right pneumothorax. There is a suggestion of a bullous lesion at the apex of the right lung. Pneumothoraces are usually visible on normal inspiratory films, but an expiratory film may help when there is doubt. There is no mediastinal displacement on examination or radiograph; movement of the mediastinum away from the side of the pneumothorax would suggest a tension pneumothorax. Although she had symptoms initially, these have settled down as might be expected in a fit patient with no underlying lung disease. A rim of air greater than 2 cm around the lung on the radiograph indicates at least a moderate pneumothorax because of the three-dimensional structure of the lung within the thoracic cage represented on the two-dimensional radiograph.

The differential diagnosis of chest pain in a young woman includes pneumonia and pleurisy, pulmonary embolism and musculoskeletal problems. However, the clinical signs and radiograph leave no doubt about the diagnosis in this woman. Pneumothoraces are more common in tall, thin men; in smokers; and in those with underlying lung disease. Further investigations such as computed tomography (CT) scan are not indicated unless there is a suggestion of underlying lung disease.

There is a suggestion that she may have had a similar episode in the past, but it may have been on the left side. There is a tendency for recurrence of pneumothoraces, between 30% and 50% will have an ipsilateral recurrent pneumothorax. Unless an intervention is undertaken, a third and fourth event can be expected in 62% and 83% of patients. Because of this, pleurodesis should be considered after two pneumothoraces or for those whose occupations might be affected, such as professional divers or pilots.

The immediate management is to aspirate the pneumothorax through the second intercostal space anteriorly using a 16–18-gauge cannula at least 3 cm long. Small pneumothoraces with no symptoms and no underlying lung disease can be left to absorb spontaneously, but this is quite a slow process. Up to 2500 mL can be aspirated at one time, stopping if it becomes difficult to aspirate or the patient coughs excessively. If the aspiration is unsuccessful or the pneumothorax recurs immediately, intercostal drainage to an underwater seal or valve may be indicated. Difficulties at this stage or a persistent air leak may require thoracic surgical intervention. This is considered earlier than it used to be since the adoption of less-invasive video-assisted techniques has become widespread. In this woman, the apical bulla was associated with a persistent leak and required minimally invasive surgical intervention through video-assisted thoracoscopic surgery.

She should be offered support to stop smoking since tobacco smoking increases the risk of recurrence of pneumothorax. Marijuana has been reported to be associated with bullous lung disease, and this patient should be advised to avoid it.

The presence of a pneumothorax is an absolute contraindication to air travel as trapped air may expand and result in a tension pneumothorax. The Civil Aviation Authority suggests patients may travel 2 weeks after successful drainage if there is no residual air. Activities such as scuba diving should be permanently avoided unless the patient has undergone bilateral surgical pleurectomy and has normal lung function and chest CT postoperatively.

🔑 **KEY POINTS**

- The patient should not be allowed to fly for at least 1 week after the pneumothorax has resolved with full expansion of the lung, confirmed on chest radiograph (2 weeks after a traumatic pneumothorax).
- The risk of recurrence will be reduced by stopping smoking.

CASE 63: EXCESSIVE DAYTIME SLEEPINESS

History

A 57-year-old male taxi driver presents to his general practitioner (GP) with excessive daytime sleepiness. For the past 2 years, he has had a tendency to fall asleep whilst he is reading, watching TV or sitting quietly. On two occasions, he has fallen asleep whilst driving. The first occurred at a traffic light. He was woken by the beeping of a car behind him. He also fell asleep whilst driving on a motorway and drifted into another lane before waking. He sleeps for 8 hours at night. He has woken up a few times gasping for air. His wife reports he is a loud snorer. On some occasions, he stops breathing and she has felt the need to prod him for him to resume breathing. He takes ramipril and bendroflumethiazide for hypertension. Overnight oximetry is performed and shown in Figure 63.1.

Examination

On examination his body mass index (BMI) is 41 kg/m². His blood pressure is 168/98 mmHg. His oropharynx is crowded and red. Tonsils are normal sized. Cardiopulmonary examination is normal.

🔍 **INVESTIGATIONS**

The results of overnight oximetry are shown in Figure 63.1.

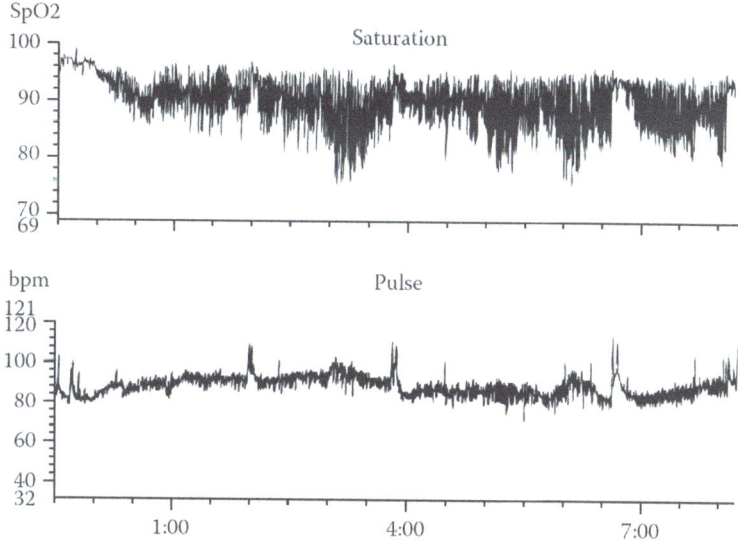

Figure 63.1 Overnight oximetry.

❓ **QUESTIONS**

- What is the diagnosis?
- What is the management of this condition?
- What advice would you give him about driving?

DOI: 10.1201/9781003350934-70

ANSWER 63

The causes of excessive daytime sleepiness include inadequate sleep opportunity, obstructive sleep apnoea (OSA), narcolepsy, periodic limb movements in sleep, depression and medication. Despite adequate sleep opportunity (>7 hours), this patient describes excessive daytime sleepiness. This patient has symptoms of OSA with snoring, nocturnal dyspnoea, witnessed apnoea and daytime sleepiness. Other symptoms of sleep apnoea include fatigue, poor concentration, nocturia, nocturnal choking, sore throat and morning headache.

OSA is due to episodic collapse of the lumen of the upper airway during sleep. It results in airflow obstruction, oxygen desaturation and arousals from sleep. The frequent arousals from sleep result in daytime somnolence. Sleep apnoea causes hypertension and is a common cause of resistant hypertension. It is also an independent risk factor for heart disease and stroke. Patients may not be aware they have sleep apnoea and present with daytime sleepiness.

Sleep studies are required to confirm OSA. In this case, an overnight oximetry shows recurrent oxygen desaturations and heart rate rises consistent with OSA. Overnight oximetry is a useful tool; however, more detailed testing, such as an inpatient polysomnography, may be required if overnight oximetry is not diagnostic. The Epworth sleepiness scale and STOP-Bang questionnaire are screening questionnaires that can be used to assess the extent and severity of symptoms, often used in community settings.

The treatment of sleep apnoea includes weight loss, mandibular advancement splints (MAS) and continuous positive airway pressure (CPAP). Tonsillectomy can be performed if tonsils are very enlarged; this is the commonest treatment of sleep apnoea in children.

CPAP is a device that provides positive airway pressure through a facemask. The positive pressure splints the upper airway open and prevents it from collapsing during sleep. CPAP is recommended for the treatment of moderate and severe OSA. Mandibular advancement splints are used in mild sleep apnoea. These are gum shields worn at night that pull the lower jaw forward and open the lumen of the airway.

Obesity is a major reversible risk factor for OSA. The increasing prevalence of obesity worldwide has been accompanied by an increase in OSA. Weight loss should be recommended for all patients with OSA who are overweight (BMI ≥25 kg/m²). Dietary advice (e.g., reduce alcohol intake), behaviour modification (e.g., avoid sleeping on their back and to sleep on their side) and regular exercise should be recommended. Bariatric surgery has a high success rate of weight loss and resolution of OSA. Bariatric surgery should be considered in patients with a BMI ≥40 kg/m² or BMI of 35–40 kg/m² with a co-morbid condition (such as diabetes mellitus, OSA or hypertension).

In most countries, OSA is a notifiable condition to the driving authorities. In the UK, this patient should not drive until treatment has started and sleepiness has resolved.

🔑 **KEY POINTS**

- There is an increasing prevalence of obesity and OSA worldwide due to obesity.
- OSA presents with excessive daytime sleepiness and is a common cause of resistant hypertension.
- Treatment of OSA is usually with CPAP and weight loss.

CASE 64: PAIN IN THE CHEST

History

A 48-year-old man presents to the emergency department with left-sided chest pain. Ten days earlier, he was unwell with a cough, shortness of breath and fever. He saw his general practitioner (GP) who prescribed amoxicillin and paracetamol. After 48 hours, he felt better and stopped taking the antibiotics.

Over the last 2 days, he has felt unwell and lost his appetite. Alongside the chest discomfort, his fever has returned. The cough has resolved but he is now short of breath on exertion.

He smokes 20 cigarettes per day and drinks 5 to 6 pints of beer most days. He is unemployed. His diet is poor and he has lost 6 kg in weight over the past year.

In his medical history he had an admission for a chest infection 6 years previously and has had treatment on and off for peptic ulceration. There is no family history of note.

Examination

He is thin. His respiratory rate is 22/min, blood pressure is 124/76, pulse is 96/min, oxygen saturation is 95% breathing air. On examination of his chest, there is some dullness to percussion with reduced breath sounds at the left base.

🔍 INVESTIGATIONS

		Normal
Haemoglobin	12.2 g/dL	11.7–15.7 g/dL
Mean corpuscular volume (MCV)	82 fL	80–99 fL
White cell count	18.9 × 10⁹/L	3.5–11.0 × 10⁹/L
Platelets	450 × 10⁹/L	150–440 × 10⁹/L
C-reactive protein (CRP)	282 mg/L	<5 mg/L

A chest radiograph is shown in Figure 64.1.

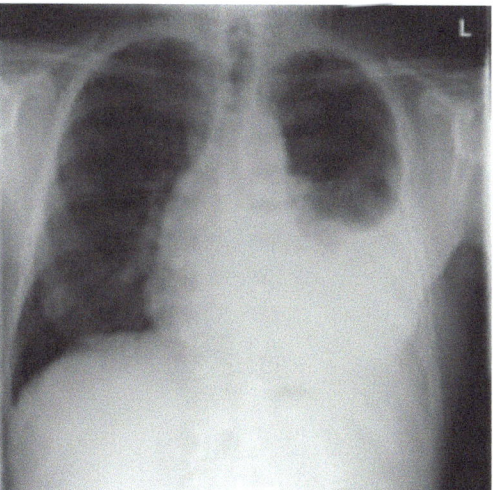

Figure 64.1 Chest radiograph.

❓ QUESTIONS

- What is the most likely diagnosis?
- How would you investigate this patient?
- How would you manage this patient?

DOI: 10.1201/9781003350934-71

ANSWER 64

The history suggests a partially treated pneumonia. The systemic symptoms, white cell count and inflammatory markers indicate infection. The chest radiograph and the clinical findings show a left pleural effusion.

Pleural effusions can occur in association with pneumonia when they may be parapneumonic effusions related to the inflammation at the pleural surface of the lung. Such effusions resolve without intervention as the pneumonia is treated. However, in this man, it is more likely that the effusion is purulent, i.e., an empyema. This needs to be established by aspiration of the fluid. This is best done under ultrasound guidance to reduce the likelihood of complications from needle aspiration.

Empyemas are more likely to develop when there is inadequate antibiotic treatment or underlying problems with immunity. In this case, antibiotics were discontinued too soon and his poor nutrition and high alcohol intake increased his risk. The most common bacterial cause of empyema is *Streptococcus pneumoniae*, though anaerobic bacteria are sometimes implicated. If risk factors are present, consider tuberculosis as a cause.

In this case, an ultrasound did reveal an effusion with echogenic debris but no loculation (where an effusion is divided into smaller compartments by fibrous septations, making them difficult to drain). Foul smelling pus was aspirated from the space using a needle. A particularly bad smell may indicate anaerobic infection. The aspirated fluid should be sent for estimation of pH, protein, glucose (with a simultaneous blood glucose test), culture and cytology (if applicable, to look for neoplastic causes). A pH <7.20 and low glucose are suggestive of an empyema.

As with any significant collection of pus, empyemas require physical drainage as well as antibiotics. An adequate-sized drain should be inserted, best placed under radiological control. If this fails to drain the fluid adequately, thoracic surgical intervention may be required to break down adhesions or loculations and ensure adequate drainage. Thrombolytic agents have been used to help drainage but a meta-analysis suggested no significant benefit on outcome.

 KEY POINTS

- Pleural effusions associated with pneumonia may be sympathetic effusions or associated infection in the pleural space.
- Pleural aspiration and drainage should be done with ultrasound guidance.
- Ensure pleural fluid is sent for microscopy, cultures, pH, protein and glucose.
- Adequate drainage for empyemas should be established as soon as possible after diagnosis.

CASE 65: COUGH AND BREATHLESSNESS

History

A 69-year-old widower smoked 20 cigarettes a day for more than 40 years but then gave them up 9 months ago when his first grandchild was born. He has had a cough with daily sputum production for the last 20 years and has become short of breath over the last 3 years. He coughs up a white to yellow shade of sputum every morning. He has put on weight recently and now weighs 100 kg. His ankles have become swollen recently and his exercise tolerance has decreased. He can no longer carry his shopping back from the supermarket 180 m (200 yards) away. He worked as a warehouseman until he was 65 and has become frustrated by his inability to do what he used to do. He is not able to look after his grandchild because he feels too short of breath.

There is no other relevant medical or family history. He lives alone and has a cat and a budgerigar at home.

His general practitioner (GP) gave him a salbutamol metered-dose inhaler, which produced no improvement in his symptoms.

Examination

He is overweight. He appears to be centrally and peripherally cyanosed and has some pitting oedema of his ankles. His jugular venous pressure is raised 3 cm. He has poor chest expansion. There are some early inspiratory crackles at the lung bases.

🔍 INVESTIGATIONS

Respiratory function test results are shown:

	Actual	Predicted
FEV$_1$ (L)	0.47	2.8–3.6
FVC (L)	1.35	3.8–4.6
FER (FEV$_1$/FVC) (%)	35	72–80
PEF (L/min)	90	310–440

Abbreviations: FEV$_1$: forced expiratory volume in 1 s; FVC: forced vital capacity; FER: forced expiratory ratio; PEF: peak expiratory flow.

His chest radiograph is shown in Figure 65.1.

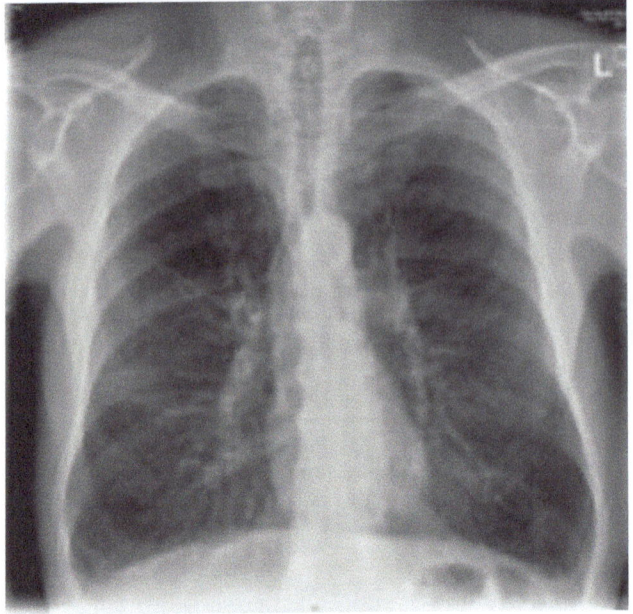

Figure 65.1 Chest radiograph.

? | **QUESTIONS**

- What does the radiograph show?
- What is the likely diagnosis?
- What management is appropriate?

ANSWER 65

The most likely diagnosis is chronic obstructive pulmonary disease (COPD). The physical signs and chest radiograph indicate overinflation. The early inspiratory crackles are typical of COPD.

Treatment with bronchodilators should be pursued. Notably, short-acting beta-2 agonists (SABAs) and short-acting muscarinic antagonists (SAMAs). Efficacy of the medication can be reported by a relief in the patient's symptoms and an improvement in their exercise tolerance. A spirometry is not required for diagnosis or treatment efficacy, but it is useful in determining the severity of the disease. Theophylline may sometimes be useful as a third-line therapy but has more side effects.

With this degree of severity (FEV_1 <50%), inhaled corticosteroids and long-acting bronchodilators (salmeterol/formoterol or tiotropium) would be appropriate inhaled therapy. Careful attention would need to be given to inhaler technique.

He is cyanosed and has signs of right-sided heart failure (*cor pulmonale*). Blood gases should be checked to see if he might be a candidate for long-term home oxygen therapy (known to improve survival if the pressure of arterial oxygen (p_aO_2) in the steady-state breathing air remains ≤7.3 kPa). Gentle diuresis might help the oedema, although oxygen would be a better approach if he is sufficiently hypoxic. Annual influenza vaccination should be recommended and *Streptococcus pneumoniae* vaccination should be given. Prophylactic antibiotics (e.g., azithromycin) might be kept at home for infective exacerbations, as part of a patient's 'rescue pack'. Patients should also be offered treatment and support to smoking cessation.

Exercise tolerance will be influenced by obesity; therefore, weight management should be discussed. Pulmonary rehabilitation is greatly valued by patients and has been shown to increase exercise tolerance by around 20% and improve quality of life. Other interventions such as lung reduction surgery or transplantation are last-line in the management of COPD and are indicated in patients with very severe airflow limitation. Depression is often associated with poor exercise tolerance and social isolation, and this should be considered.

COPD is often regarded as a condition for which treatment has little to offer. However, a vigorous approach tailored to the needs of the individual patient can provide a worthwhile benefit.

🔑 KEY POINTS

- In COPD, beta-2 agonists and anticholinergic agents produce similar effects or a greater response from anticholinergics. The combination may be helpful. In contrast, in asthma, beta-2 agonists produce a greater effect.
- Assessment for home oxygen should be made in a stable state on optimal inhaled therapy.
- Exercise and diet are important elements in the management of COPD.
- Depression is common in chronic conditions such as COPD.

CASE 66: SHORTNESS OF BREATH

History

A 35-year-old woman presents with a 6-month history of increasing shortness of breath. This has progressed so that she is now short of breath on walking up one flight of stairs and walks more slowly on the flat than other people her age. In addition, she has developed a dry cough over the past 3 months.

Her past medical history includes having mild asthma as a child. She thinks that her father died of a chest problem in his 40s. She takes occasional paracetamol and has taken 'slimming pills' in the past.

She is a lifetime non-smoker and drinks less than 10 units of alcohol per week. She has worked in the printing trade since she left school. She has two children, aged 8 and 10 years, and they have a cat and a rabbit at home.

Examination

There is no clubbing, anaemia or cyanosis. Examination of the cardiovascular system is normal. In the respiratory system, expansion of the lungs seems to be reduced but symmetrical. The percussion note is normal, as is tactile vocal fremitus. On auscultation, there are some fine late inspiratory crackles at both lung bases.

 INVESTIGATIONS

Respiratory function tests revealed the following:

	Actual	Predicted
FEV_1 (L)	3.0	3.6–4.2
FVC (L)	3.6	4.5–5.3
FER (FEV_1/FVC) (%)	83	75–80
PEF (L/min)	470	450–550

Abbreviations: FEV_1: forced expiratory volume in 1 s; FVC: forced vital capacity; FER: forced expiratory ratio; PEF: peak expiratory flow.

Her chest radiograph is shown in Figure 66.1 and a high-resolution computed tomography (CT) scan in Figure 66.2.

DOI: 10.1201/9781003350934-73

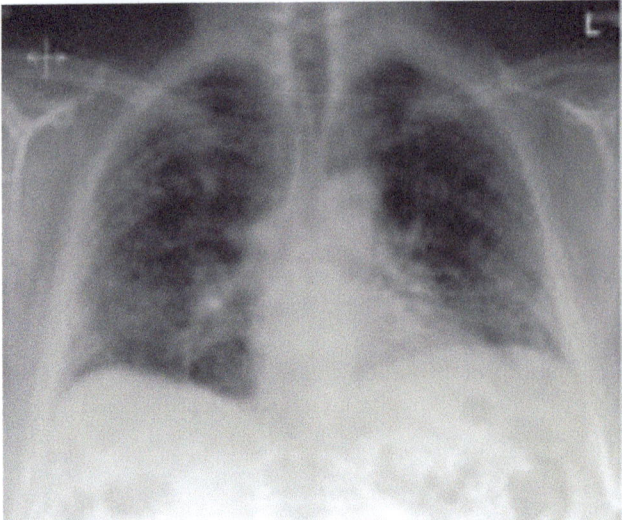

Figure 66.1 Chest radiograph.

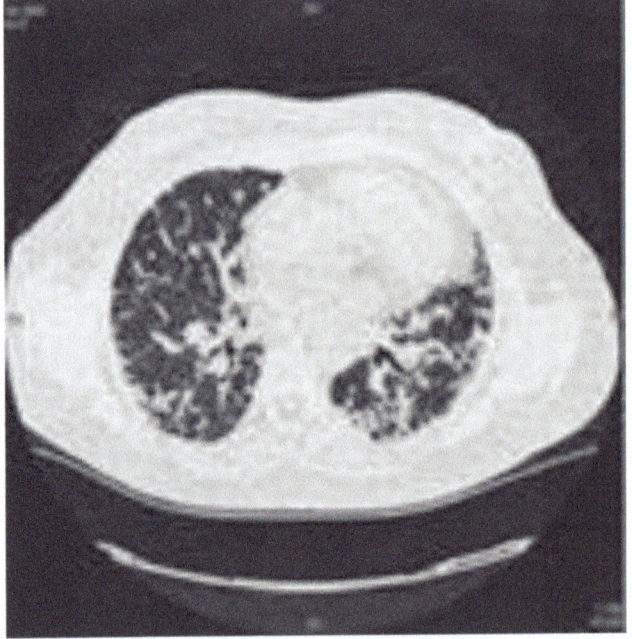

Figure 66.2 High-resolution computed tomography scan.

? QUESTIONS

- What is the likely diagnosis?
- What further investigations are indicated?
- What treatment options are there?

ANSWER 66

The history shows a progressive condition over at least 6 months. It is often difficult to be sure of the exact length of history when a symptom such as breathlessness has an insidious onset. A few possibilities are raised by the details of the history. There is a history of asthma, but the absence of wheezing or obstruction on the respiratory function tests rule that out as the cause of the current problem. An occupational history is always important in lung disease but probably not here. Occupational asthma can be associated with isocyanates used in the printing trade, but this would cause an obstructive problem rather than the restrictive problem shown here. The findings on examination fit with a restrictive problem with limited expansion and crackles caused by reopening of airways closing during expiration because of stiff lungs and low lung volumes.

The respiratory function tests show a mild restrictive ventilatory defect with reduced FEV_1 and FVC but a slightly high ratio, suggesting stiff lungs or chest wall. Further tests such as transfer factor would be expected to be reduced in the presence of pulmonary fibrosis.

The chest radiograph shows small lung fields and nodular and reticular shadowing most marked in mid- and lower zones. The high-resolution CT scan shows widespread fibrotic change with subpleural cyst formation. These changes are compatible with diffuse pulmonary fibrosis (fibrosing alveolitis). When considering fibrosis of the lungs, it is important to differentiate diffuse pulmonary fibrosis, as is the case here, and localised pulmonary fibrosis as a result of scarring after an acute inflammatory condition, such as pneumonia. The distribution and the pattern of the changes on the CT scan are important in determining the diagnosis and the likelihood of response to treatment in pulmonary fibrosis. Diffuse pulmonary fibrosis can be associated with conditions such as rheumatoid arthritis and can be induced by inhaled dusts or ingested drugs. None of these seem likely here, making this likely to be idiopathic pulmonary fibrosis (IPF). There is a rare familial form, so the father's illness might be relevant. The most common type of IPF is usual interstitial pneumonia (UIP) with a subpleural distribution, as shown on the CT scan. In association with connective tissue disease, there may be a more widespread patchy pattern of non-specific interstitial pneumonitis (NSIP). The appearance of 'ground-glass' shadowing on the high-resolution CT is associated with active cellular alveolitis and a greater likelihood of response to treatment. NSIP also has a better response rate than UIP.

Further investigations consist of a search for a cause or associated conditions and a decision whether a lung biopsy is required. Bronchoscopic biopsies are too small to be representative or useful in this situation. A video-assisted thoracoscopic biopsy would be the usual procedure. It would usually be appropriate to obtain histology of the lung in someone of this age.

Treatment mainly consists of pulmonary rehabilitation, including exercise and educational components tailored to the needs of people with IPF, and supportive care e.g., symptom relief and optimising co-morbidities. There is currently no conclusive evidence to support the use of drugs such as steroids and immunosuppressants, e.g., azathioprine, in IPF. However, there is some evidence that antioxidants such as N-acetylcysteine and antifibrotic agents like pirfenidone could improve the outlook, and new agents are under investigation. In a patient of this age, lung transplantation might be a consideration as the disease progresses. Progression rates are variable, and an acute aggressive form with death in 6 months can occur. More common in UIP is steady progression over a few years.

🔑 KEY POINTS

- Diffuse pulmonary fibrosis has a range of causes relevant to management.
- Ineffective treatment may produce serious side effects without significant benefit.

CASE 67: SHORTNESS OF BREATH

History

A 20-year-old woman has complained of intermittent shortness of breath with wheezing and cough for 3 years. She had eczema and rhinitis up to the age of 8. A diagnosis of asthma was made, but control of her symptoms has been difficult, and she is now being treated with salbutamol, salmeterol, high-dose inhaled corticosteroids and montelukast. The breathlessness is intermittent. When the breathlessness comes on, she feels unable to take air into her lung, is often unable to speak and finds that multiple doses of salbutamol provide little relief. She presents to the emergency department with an acute exacerbation of her breathlessness.

Examination

She is unable to speak in more than a whisper. Her respiratory rate is 26/min. Pulse rate is 92/min and blood pressure 128/84 mmHg. Her temperature is 36.8°C and oxygen saturation is 98% on air. The heart sounds are normal. There is a generalised inspiratory and expiratory wheeze heard all over the chest but no other abnormalities. She finds it difficult to perform a peak flow recording but manages 60 L/min.

 INVESTIGATIONS

After recovery from this acute episode, she is sent for respiratory function tests which show:

	Actual	Postbronchodilator	Predicted
FEV$_1$ (L)	3.5	3.7	3.5–4.3
FVC (L)	4.6	4.8	4.6–5.4
FER (FEV$_1$/FVC) (%)	76	77	72–80
PEF (L/min)	440	480	440–540

Abbreviations: FEV$_1$: forced expiratory volume in 1 s; FVC: forced vital capacity; FER: forced expiratory ratio; PEF: peak expiratory flow.

 QUESTIONS

- What is the most likely diagnosis?
- What further investigations are indicated?
- What treatment options are there?

DOI: 10.1201/9781003350934-74

ANSWER 67

This woman has intermittent breathlessness with wheezing. The commonest cause of these symptoms would be asthma, but there are several features which make this less likely in this patient. Loss of voice is a prominent symptom. The history suggests little response to beta agonist treatment, and the lung function tests after recovery from the episode do not show airflow obstruction or a significant response to bronchodilators. The airway narrowing in asthma may be intermittent showing no obstruction between attacks, thus it may be necessary to look for increased bronchial responsiveness to a challenge such as exercise or inhaled methacholine.

During the acute episode, in association with severe symptoms, the oxygen saturation is, surprisingly, normal. Inability to speak in complete sentences is a characteristic of severe asthma, but the loss of voice here suggests that there may be a problem at the vocal cord level and this would fit with the marked inspiratory and expiratory wheezing and the feeling of being unable to take air into her lungs, although asthmatics may complain of similar problems. These features suggest a more likely diagnosis of vocal cord dysfunction in this woman. In this condition, there is paradoxical motion of the vocal cords so that they adduct on inspiration to produce inspiratory airflow obstruction at the level of the larynx. Episodes of breathlessness tend to be intermittent, unresponsive to conventional asthma treatment and associated with stridor.

The most important diagnostic tests are direct viewing of the cords by an ear, nose and throat surgeon and a flow-volume loop. Inspection of the cords will show paradoxical motion and adduction of the anterior cords with a posterior 'glottis chink' allowing limited airflow. A flow-volume loop will show a relatively normal expiratory phase, but low or loss of flow in the latter part of the inspiratory loop as the vocal cords adduct and produce obstruction (Figure 67.1). In asthma, obstruction is evident in both expiratory and inspiratory limbs of the flow volume loop.

It is important to recognise this condition so that inappropriate treatment for asthma can be stopped and appropriate treatment can be started. Vocal cord dysfunction is present in about 10% of patients with refractory asthma. It is more common in the presence of psychiatric problems such as depression and anxiety, and may be associated with gastro-oesophageal reflux. The mainstays of treatment involve identifying and controlling triggers for these episodes, speech therapy, relaxation and breathing techniques.

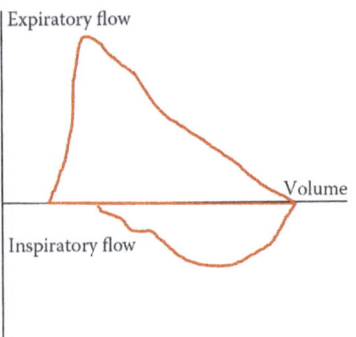

Figure 67.1 Flow–volume loop showing cutoff of inspiratory flow in vocal cord dysfunction.

🔑 **KEY POINTS**

- When asthma is difficult to control, other diagnoses such as vocal cord dysfunction or large airway obstruction should be considered.
- Flow-volume loops may be useful in differentiating causes of airflow obstruction.

Section 8
NEPHROLOGY

CASE 68: TIREDNESS

History

An 85-year-old woman is investigated by her general practitioner (GP) for increasing tiredness, which has developed over the past 6 months. She has lost her appetite and feels constantly nauseated. She has lost about 8 kg in weight over the past 6 months. For the last 4 weeks, she has also complained of generalised itching and cramps. She has been hypertensive for 20 years and has been on antihypertensive medication for that time. She has had two cerebrovascular accidents, which have left her with some left-side weakness and reduced mobility. She is of African-Caribbean origin, having emigrated to the United Kingdom in the 1960s. She lives alone but uses a 'meals-on-wheels' service and goes to a day hospital twice a week. She has two daughters.

Examination

Her conjunctivae are pale. Her pulse is 88/min regular, blood pressure 190/110 mmHg; mild pitting oedema of her ankles is present. Otherwise, examination of her cardiovascular and respiratory systems is normal. Neurological examination shows a left upper motor neurone facial palsy with mild weakness and increased tone and reflexes in the left arm and leg. She is able to walk with a stick. Fundoscopy shows arteriovenous nipping and increased tortuosity of the arteries.

🔍 INVESTIGATIONS

		Normal
Haemoglobin	7.8 g/dL	11.7–15.7 g/dL
Mean corpuscular volume (MCV)	84 fL	80–99 fL
White cell count	6.3×10^9/L	$3.5–11.0 \times 10^9$/L
Platelets	294×10^9/L	$150–440 \times 10^9$/L
Sodium	136 mmol/L	135–145 mmol/L
Potassium	4.8 mmol/L	3.5–5.0 mmol/L
Urea	46.2 mmol/L	2.5–6.7 mmol/L
Creatinine	769 µmol/L	70–120 µmol/L
Glucose	4.4 mmol/L	4.0–6.0 mmol/L
Albumin	37 g/L	35–50 g/L
Calcium	1.94 mmol/L	2.12–2.65 mmol/L
Phosphate	3.4 mmol/L	0.8–1.45 mmol/L
Bilirubin	15 mmol/L	3–17 mmol/L
Alanine transaminase	23 IU/L	5–35 IU/L
Alkaline phosphatase	423 IU/L	30–300 IU/L

Urinalysis: 1 protein; 1 blood

Blood film: normochromic, normocytic anaemia

❓ QUESTIONS

- What is the diagnosis?
- What investigations are indicated for this patient?
- How would you manage this patient?

DOI: 10.1201/9781003350934-76

ANSWER 68

This patient presents anorexia, nausea, weight loss, fatigue, pruritus and cramps. These are typical symptoms of end-stage kidney failure.

The elevated urea and creatinine levels confirm renal failure but do not distinguish between acute and chronic renal failure. Usually, in the former, there is evidence of either a systemic illness or some other obvious precipitating cause (e.g., use of nephrotoxic drugs/prolonged episode of hypotension), whereas in the latter, there is a prolonged history of general malaise. If the patient has had previous blood tests measuring serum creatinine, these will be informative about the progression of deterioration of renal function. In this patient, the anaemia and hyperparathyroidism (raised alkaline phosphatase) are features indicating chronicity of the renal failure. The normochromic normocytic anaemia is predominantly due to erythropoietin deficiency (the kidney is the major source of erythropoietin production). Urinalysis positive for blood and protein excreted in urine are pathological markers for kidney damage. Urinary albumin measures based on albumin excretion rate or albumin creatinine ratio (moderately increased albuminuria) can reflect the progression of chronic renal failure associated with hypertension or diabetes mellitus.

Hyperparathyroidism is a result of elevated serum phosphate levels due to decreased renal clearance of phosphate and reduced vitamin D levels (the kidney is the site of hydroxylation of 25-hydroxycholecalciferol to the active form 1,25-dihydroxycholecalciferol). A hand radiograph shows the typical appearances of hyperparathyroidism (erosion of the terminal phalanges and subperiosteal erosions of the radial aspects of the middle phalanges).

Renal ultrasound is the essential investigation. Ultrasound will accurately size the kidneys and identify obvious causes for renal failure, such as polycystic kidney disease or obstruction causing bilateral hydronephrosis. Asymmetrically sized kidneys suggest reflux nephropathy or renovascular disease. In this case, ultrasound showed two small (8 cm) echogenic kidneys consistent with long-standing renal failure. A renal biopsy in this case is not appropriate as biopsies of small kidneys have a high incidence of bleeding complications, and the sample obtained would show extensive glomerular and tubulointerstitial fibrosis and may not identify the original disease. The patient's renal failure may have been due to hypertension or a primary glomerulonephritis such as immunoglobulin A (IgA) nephropathy. Patients of African-Caribbean origin are more prone to develop hypertensive renal failure than other racial groups.

Antihypertensive medications are needed to treat her blood pressure adequately, oral phosphate binders and vitamin D preparations to control her secondary hyperparathyroidism and erythropoietin injections to treat her anaemia. Serial blood serum assessments determine calcium, phosphate and PTH levels. The case raises the dilemma of whether dialysis is appropriate in this patient. Hospital-based haemodialysis and home-based peritoneal dialysis are the options available. Her age and comorbid illnesses preclude renal transplantation. Conservative management without dialysis may be appropriate in this case.

 KEY POINTS

- Patients often become symptomatic due to renal failure only when their glomerular filtration rate (GFR) is less than 15 mL/min and thus may present with end-stage renal failure.
- Renal replacement therapy initiated in patients with uraemia signs such as hyperkalaemia, acidosis, fluid overload, weight loss, appetite loss, nausea and vomiting.
- Previous measurements of serum creatinine enable the rate of deterioration of renal function to be known.
- Renal ultrasound is the key imaging investigation.

CASE 69: BACK PAIN

History

A 27-year-old woman attends the emergency department complaining of left-sided back pain. She became unwell 2 days ago with a fever and a dull back ache. The pain is increasing in severity. She has vomited twice in the past 6 hours. She has no significant medical history apart from an uncomplicated episode of cystitis 3 months ago.

Examination

She looks unwell and is flushed. Her temperature is 39.5°C. Her pulse is 120/min and blood pressure is 104/68 mmHg. Examination of the cardiovascular and respiratory systems is unremarkable. Her abdomen is generally tender, but most markedly in both loins. Bowel sounds are normal.

🔍 INVESTIGATIONS

		Normal
Haemoglobin	15.3 g/dL	11.7–15.7 g/dL
White cell count	25.2 × 10⁹/L	3.5–11.0 × 10⁹/L
Platelets	406 × 10⁹/L	150–440 × 10⁹/L
Sodium	134 mmol/L	135–145 mmol/L
Potassium	4.1 mmol/L	3.5–5.0 mmol/L
Urea	14.2 mmol/L	2.5–6.7 mmol/L
Creatinine	106 µmol/L	70–120 µmol/L
Albumin	44 g/L	35–50 g/L
C-reactive protein (CRP)	316 mg/L	<5 mg/L

Urinalysis: protein +; blood +++; leucocytes ++; nitrites positive
Urine microscopy: >50 red cells; >50 white cells
Abdominal radiograph: normal

? QUESTIONS

- What is the likely diagnosis?
- What investigations are indicated for this patient?
- How would you manage this patient?

ANSWER 69

This woman has symptoms and signs of acute pyelonephritis. Pyelonephritis is more common in women and occurs when bacteria ascend and infect the upper urinary tract. Pregnancy, diabetes mellitus, immunosuppression and structurally abnormal urinary tracts are risk factors for ascending infection.

> **! DIFFERENTIAL DIAGNOSIS**
>
> **Pyelonephritis** causes loin pain, which can be unilateral or bilateral. The differential diagnosis of loin pain includes **obstructive uropathy, renal infarction, renal cell carcinoma, renal papillary necrosis, renal calculi, glomerulonephritis, polycystic kidney disease, medullary sponge kidney** and **loin-pain haematuria syndrome**.

Fever may be as high as 40°C with associated systemic symptoms of anorexia, nausea and vomiting. Some patients may have preceding symptoms of cystitis (dysuria, urinary frequency, urgency and haematuria) or report an episode of cystitis in the prior 6 months, but these lower urinary tract symptoms may not always occur. Elderly patients may present with non-specific symptoms and confusion.

Pyelonephritis may also mimic other conditions, such as acute appendicitis, acute cholecystitis, acute pancreatitis and lower lobe pneumonia. There is usually marked tenderness over the kidneys both posteriorly and anteriorly (costovertebral tenderness). Untreated infection may lead to septic shock.

The raised white cell count and CRP are consistent with an acute bacterial infection. Microscopic haematuria, proteinuria and leucocytes in the urine suggest inflammation in the urinary tract. The presence of bacteria in the urine is confirmed by the reduction of nitrates to nitrites.

This woman requires admission. Blood and urine cultures should be collected prior to empirical intravenous antibiotics, prescribed according to local guidance. Once the bacteria and their sensitivities are identified, she can be switched to a narrow spectrum antibiotic. An example of empirical therapy is gentamicin with cefuroxime or amoxicillin-clavulanic acid. Intravenous fluids, antipyretics and antiemetics are prescribed as needed. If she is slow to respond to antibiotics, a renal ultrasound scan should be performed to exclude complications such as renal abscess formation or pus collecting in the kidney (pyonephrosis), which may require drainage.

Patients with an uncomplicated renal infection should be treated with a minimum 7 days of antibiotics, but this can be extended depending on clinical response. In patients with infection complicated by stones, or where there is urological obstruction, involvement of the urology and microbiology teams is essential.

> **⚷ KEY POINTS**
>
> - Acute pyelonephritis may present with or without preceding lower urinary tract symptoms.
> - Urine and blood cultures should be collected and empirical antibiotics started (usually consisting of two separate classes e.g., an aminoglycoside and a beta-lactam) whilst cultures are awaited.
> - For patients who are slow to respond to antibiotics or whose condition worsens on treatment, a renal ultrasound should be sought to look for complications such as abscess formation or whether there is obstruction.

CASE 70: ANKLE SWELLING

History

A 72-year-old man goes to his general practitioner (GP) complaining of painless swelling of both legs, which he first noted approximately 2 months ago. The swelling started at the ankles, but now his legs, thighs and genitals are swollen. His face is puffy in the mornings on getting up. His weight is up by about 10 kg over the previous 3 months. He has noticed that his urine appears to be frothy in the toilet. He has noted gradual increasing shortness of breath but denies any chest pain. He has also developed spontaneous bruising over the past 6 months. He is a retired heavy goods vehicle driver. He had hypertension diagnosed 13 years ago and a myocardial infarction 4 years previously. He lives with his wife and has no children. He continues to smoke 30 cigarettes a day and drinks about 30 units of alcohol a week. His medication consists of atenolol 50 mg once a day.

Examination

On examination, there is pitting oedema of the legs, which is present to the level of the sacrum. There is also massive oedema of the penis and scrotum. There is bruising on the forearms and around the eyes. There are no signs of chronic liver disease. His pulse rate is 72/min and regular. Blood pressure is 166/78 mmHg. His jugular venous pressure is raised at 5 cm. His apex beat is not displaced, and auscultation reveals normal heart sounds and no murmurs. There is dullness to percussion and reduced air entry at both lung bases. The liver, spleen and kidneys are not palpable, but ascites is demonstrated by shifting dullness and fluid thrill. Neurological examination is unremarkable.

🔍 INVESTIGATIONS

		Normal
Haemoglobin	10.7 g/dL	13.3–17.7 g/dL
Mean corpuscular volume (MCV)	95 fL	80–99 fL
White cell count	4.7×10^9/L	3.9–10.6×10^9/L
Platelets	176×10^9/L	150–440×10^9/L
Sodium	138 mmol/L	135–145 mmol/L
Potassium	4.9 mmol/L	3.5–5.0 mmol/L
Urea	7.4 mmol/L	2.5–6.7 mmol
Creatinine	112 μmol/L	70–120 μmol/L
Glucose	4.7 mmol/L	4.0–6.0 mmol/L
Albumin	16 g/L	35–50 g/L
Cholesterol	15.2 mmol/L	3.9–6.0 mmol/L
Triglycerides	2.7 mmol/L	0.55–1.90 mmol/L

Clotting screen: normal
Urinalysis: +++ protein; no blood

❓ QUESTIONS

- What is the cause of this patient's oedema?
- What is the likely underlying diagnosis?
- How would you further examine, investigate and manage this patient?

DOI: 10.1201/9781003350934-78

ANSWER 70

Peripheral oedema may occur due to local obstruction of lymphatic or venous outflow or because of cardiac, renal, pulmonary or liver disease. Unilateral oedema is most likely to be due to a local problem, whereas bilateral leg oedema is usually due to one of the medical conditions listed. Pitting oedema needs to be distinguished from lymphoedema, which is characteristically non-pitting. This is tested by firm pressure with the thumb for approximately 10 s. If the oedema is pitting, an indentation will be present after pressure is removed. This man has a subacute onset of massive pitting oedema. The major differential diagnoses are cardiac failure, renal failure, nephrotic syndrome, right heart failure (*cor pulmonale*) secondary to chronic obstructive airways disease or decompensated chronic liver disease. The frothy urine is a clue to the diagnosis of nephrotic syndrome and is commonly noted by patients with heavy proteinuria.

On examination, there were no clinical signs to suggest chronic liver disease. The jugular venous pressure would be expected to be increased more, and there should have been signs of tricuspid regurgitation (prominent 'v' wave, pansystolic murmur loudest on inspiration) and cardiomegaly if the patient had *cor pulmonale* or biventricular cardiac failure. The patient has signs of bilateral pleural effusions, which may occur in nephrotic syndrome if there is sufficient fluid retention. The bruising and periorbital purpura are classically seen in patients with nephrotic syndrome secondary to amyloidosis.

The investigations are consistent with the diagnosis of nephrotic syndrome. Nephrotic syndrome is defined by the triad of hypoalbuminaemia (<30 g/L), proteinuria (>3 g/24 h) and hyperlipidaemia. Normochromic normocytic anaemia is typical of chronic disease and is a clue to the underlying diagnosis of amyloidosis. Patients with amyloidosis may have raised serum transaminase levels due to liver infiltration by amyloid.

The patient should have a renal biopsy to delineate the cause of the nephrotic syndrome. The principal causes of nephrotic syndrome are listed below. Adults presenting with nephrotic syndrome should have a renal biopsy. The exception is the patient with long-standing diabetes mellitus, with concomitant retinopathy and neuropathy, who almost certainly has diabetic nephropathy.

> **! CAUSES OF NEPHROTIC SYNDROME**
>
> - Diabetes mellitus
> - Minimal change disease
> - Focal and segmental glomerulosclerosis
> - Membranous nephropathy
> - Systemic lupus erythematosus
> - Human immunodeficiency virus (HIV) infection
> - Plasma cell dyscrasias

In this case, renal biopsy confirmed the diagnosis of amyloidosis, and staining was positive for lambda light chains. Immunofixation confirmed the presence of IgG lambda paraprotein in the blood. Positive apple-green birefringence when biopsy specimen tested with Congo-red staining. A bone marrow aspirate showed the presence of an excessive number of plasma cells, consistent with an underlying plasma cell dyscrasia. Patients with amyloidosis should have an echocardiogram to screen for cardiac infiltration, and if the facilities are available, a serum amyloid P scan should be arranged, which assesses the distribution and total body burden of amyloid. An amyloid P scan is shown in Figure 70.1.

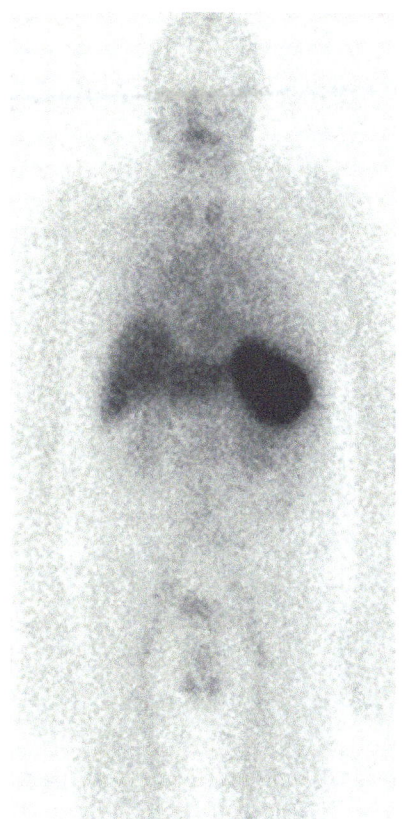

Figure 70.1 Serum amyloid P scan showing uptake predominantly in the spleen.

The initial treatment of this patient involves fluid and salt restriction and diuretics to reduce the oedema. He should be anticoagulated to reduce the risk of deep vein thrombosis or pulmonary embolus. His hyperlipidaemia should be treated with a statin. Definitive treatment is by chemotherapy supervised by the haematologists to suppress the amyloidogenic plasma cell clone. In younger patients, bone marrow transplantation may be considered. Patients with nephrotic syndrome secondary to amyloidosis usually progress to end-stage renal failure relatively quickly. Death is most commonly due to cardiac involvement.

 KEY POINTS

- Bilateral oedema may be due to cardiac, liver or renal disease.
- All patients presenting with new-onset oedema should have a urinalysis.
- Patients with nephrotic syndrome are at increased risk of pulmonary embolism.

CASE 71: HIGH BLOOD PRESSURE

History

A 36-year-old woman is referred by her general practitioner (GP) to a hypertension clinic. She was noted to be hypertensive when she joined the practice 2 years previously. Her blood pressure has been difficult to control, and she is currently taking four agents (bendroflumethiazide, atenolol, amlodipine and doxazosin). She had normal blood pressure and no pre-eclampsia during her only pregnancy 9 years previously. There is no family history of premature hypertension. She smokes 20 cigarettes a day and drinks less than 10 units a week. She is not on an oral contraceptive pill. She works part-time as a teaching assistant.

Examination

She is not overweight and looks well. Her pulse rate is 68/min and blood pressure is 180/102 mmHg. There is no radiofemoral delay. There are no café-au-lait spots or neurofibromas. Examination of the cardiovascular, respiratory and abdominal systems is normal. The fundi show no significant changes of hypertension.

🔍 INVESTIGATIONS

		Normal
Haemoglobin	13.3 g/dL	11.7–15.7 g/dL
White cell count	6.2×10^9/L	3.5–11.0×10^9/L
Platelets	266×10^9/L	150–440×10^9/L
Sodium	139 mmol/L	135–145 mmol/L
Potassium	4.4 mmol/L	3.5–5.0 mmol/L
Urea	10.7 mmol/L	2.5–6.7 mmol/L
Creatinine	136 µmol/L	70–120 µmol/L
Albumin	42 g/L	35–50 g/L

Urinalysis: no protein; no blood

Renal ultrasound: normal-size kidneys

Results of a renal angiogram are shown in Figure 71.1.

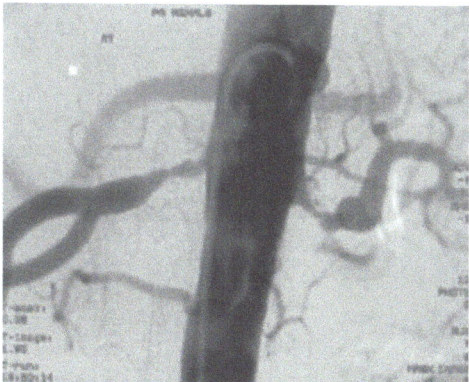

Figure 71.1 Renal angiogram.

❓ QUESTIONS

- What is the diagnosis?
- What are the main risk factors for this patient?
- What would be the appropriate management of this patient?

DOI: 10.1201/9781003350934-79

ANSWER 71

This woman has hypertension due to renovascular disease. The great majority of cases of hypertension are due to essential hypertension. Risk factors for essential hypertension include a family history of hypertension, obesity and lack of exercise. She does not have paroxysmal symptoms of sweating, palpitations and anxiety to suggest a phaeochromocytoma. There are no clinical features to suggest coarctation of the aorta (*radiofemoral delay*) or neurofibromatosis (café-au-lait spots/neurofibromas). Serum potassium is not low even on thiazide treatment, making Conn's syndrome or Cushing's syndrome unlikely. The principal abnormality is the modestly raised creatinine, suggesting mildly impaired renal function. The absence of haematuria and proteinuria excludes glomerulonephritis. Therefore, renovascular disease needs to be considered. The absence of a renal bruit on auscultation of the abdomen does not exclude the possibility of renovascular disease. The renal angiogram shows bilateral fibromuscular dysplasia (FMD).

The commonest cause of renovascular disease is atherosclerotic renal artery stenosis (ARAS). This is common in elderly patients with evidence of generalised atherosclerosis (peripheral vascular disease and coronary artery disease). Ultrasound will often show small kidneys, and renal impairment is common. ARAS is a common cause of end-stage renal failure in the elderly.

At this woman's age, atherosclerotic renovascular disease is very unlikely. FMD is the second commonest cause of renovascular disease. The commonest form is medial fibroplasia, with thinning of the intima and media leading to formation of aneurysms alternating with stenoses, presenting the classic 'string-of-beads' appearance on angiography. It predominantly affects young and middle-aged women, with a peak incidence in the fourth decade of life. Cigarette smoking is a risk factor. FMD usually presents with hypertension but can rarely present with 'flash' pulmonary oedema. FMD can also affect the carotid arteries, causing a variety of neurological symptoms e.g., ischaemic stroke.

Treatment is with percutaneous transluminal renal angioplasty along with blood pressure control with angiotensin-converting enzyme inhibitor. Unlike atheromatous renovascular disease, the hypertension in FMD cases is often cured, leading to complete cessation of blood pressure medication. Restenosis is rare. Antiplatelets may be used if the patient is at risk of a stroke.

 KEY POINTS

- FMD is an important cause of hypertension in young and middle-aged women.
- Renal artery angioplasty will improve or even cure hypertension in many patients with FMD.
- FMD is a very rare cause of end-stage renal failure.

CASE 72: SHORTNESS OF BREATH AND REDUCED URINE OUTPUT

History

A 73-year-old woman presents to the emergency department complaining of increasing breathlessness over the previous 4 days. She had felt unwell for 2 months and has lost 4 kg in weight. She has had frequent nosebleeds, and over the past few days, has coughed up small amounts of fresh blood. She notices that she has been passing less urine in the past few days. She has no significant past medical history.

Examination

On examination, she is febrile (38°C), centrally cyanosed and looks unwell. She has a purpuric rash over her ankles. Her pulse is 104/min and blood pressure is 160/100 mmHg. Her jugular venous pressure is not raised. Her heart sounds are normal with no added sounds. Her respiratory rate is 30 breaths/min, expansion is reduced, percussion and tactile vocal fremitus are normal, but she has coarse inspiratory crackles throughout both lung fields. Her abdominal and neurological examination is normal.

🔍 INVESTIGATIONS

		Normal
Haemoglobin	10.1 g/dL	11.7–15.7 g/dL
Mean corpuscular volume (MCV)	87 fL	80–99 fL
White cell count	17.2×10^9/L	$3.9–11.0 \times 10^9$/L
Platelets	540×10^9/L	$150–440 \times 10^9$/L
Sodium	137 mmol/L	135–145 mmol/L
Potassium	6.6 mmol/L	3.5–5.0 mmol/L
Urea	45.1 mmol/L	2.5–6.7 mmol/L
Creatinine	832 µmol/L	70–120 µmol/L
Albumin	32 g/L	35–50 g/L
Calcium	2.23 mmol/L	2.12–2.65 mmol/L
Phosphate	1.9 mmol/L	0.8–1.4 mmol/L
C-reactive protein (CRP)	323 mg/L	<5 mg/L
Arterial blood gases on air:		
pH	7.18	7.38–7.44
pCO_2	5.1 kPa	4.7–6.0 kPa
pO_2	6.4 kPa	12.0–14.5 kPa

Urinalysis: ++ protein; +++ blood

Electrocardiogram (ECG): sinus tachycardia

❓ QUESTIONS

- What is the likely diagnosis?
- How would you investigate this patient?
- How would you manage this patient?

DOI: 10.1201/9781003350934-80

ANSWER 72

This patient has respiratory and renal failure. Respiratory failure may occur due to fluid over-load in renal failure, but the findings on examination (normal jugular venous pressure, coarse pan-inspiratory crackles rather than fine, late inspiratory crackles) do not support this. The chest radiograph shows bilateral infiltrates. The purpuric rash and the raised platelet count and CRP are typical of active vasculitis. Alveolar haemorrhage may produce hypoxia and radiographic shadowing without gross haemoptysis. Elevated serum creatinine, positive urinalysis for haema-turia and proteinuria are pathological indicators for renal involvement.

Major causes of pulmonary/renal syndrome are:

- **Systemic vasculitis:** Granulomatosis with polyangiitis (GPA), or Wegner's, is a vasculitis of the medium and small arteries producing a granulomatous inflamma-tion of the upper and lower respiratory tracts and a necrotising glomerulonephritis. Microscopic polyarteritis primarily affects the venules, capillaries and arterioles and can cause pulmonary haemorrhage and a similar renal lesion. Patients with both dis-eases usually have antineutrophilic cytoplasmic antibodies (ANCA).
- **Antiglomerular basement membrane disease:** Goodpasture's disease
- **Systemic lupus erythematosus**

The history of nosebleeds, implying upper respiratory tract involvement, suggests that the most likely diagnosis is GPA granulomatosis with polyangiitis (Wegener's) rather than microscopic polyarteritis. Both are conditions of small vessel vasculitis and cause necrotising glomerulone-phritis and pulmonary haemorrhage, and can affect other organs such as the skin, joints, eyes and nervous system. Anti-glomerular basement membrane disease does not cause a rash. The other principal differential diagnoses of vasculitis include atheroembolic disease, infective endo-carditis and meningococcal septicaemia.

This woman needs emergency treatment for her respiratory failure, metabolic acidosis and hyperkalaemia. She requires oxygen and may require non-invasive or mechanical ventilation. Her hyperkalaemia needs emergency treatment with intravenous calcium gluconate and an infusion of dextrose and insulin until dialysis or haemofiltration is organised.

All patients with acute renal failure should have a renal ultrasound to size the kidneys and rule out obstruction. A renal biopsy in this patient will provide histological confirmation of systemic vasculitis by showing a focal necrotising glomerulonephritis usually with crescent formation. Biopsy of nasal lesions is often unproductive, showing only necrotic tissue and may delay diagno-sis. Blood should be sent for ANCAs, which are present in about 90% of untreated cases of small vessel vasculitis. In the case of GPA, cytoplasmic ANCA (c-ANCA) are more commonly found. Her gas transfer factor will be temporarily increased because of her pulmonary haemorrhage. Computed tomography (CT) chest imaging, indicated in all patients with suspected disease, may show findings of pulmonary infiltrates, lung nodules and cavitation.

The specific treatment for this woman is high-dose immunosuppression with corticosteroids and cyclophosphamide. Rituximab is increasingly used as an alternative to cyclophosphamide in remission induction due to less toxic side effects. Plasma exchange may be considered in patients with severe organ involvement such as pulmonary-renal syndrome. However, this option carries significant risk of morbidity, including serious infection, haemodynamic instability and electro-lyte disturbance. After the acute phase, maintenance treatment is with prednisolone and a low-dose rituximab. Methotrexate (with folic acid) or azathioprine are equally effective for remission maintenance alongside a corticosteroid.

 KEY POINTS

- Clinical symptoms of GPA affecting the lungs are cough, breathlessness and haemoptysis.
- ANCAs are present in more than 90% of cases of GPA, causing pulmonary/renal involvement.
- Rapid treatment is essential to prevent irreversible tissue necrosis.

CASE 73: POSTOPERATIVE DETERIORATION

History

The medical team is asked to review a postoperative surgical patient. A 62-year-old woman had been admitted 10 days previously to have a right hemicolectomy performed for a caecal carcinoma. This was discovered on colonoscopy, which was performed to investigate iron-deficiency anaemia and change in bowel habit. She is otherwise fit with no significant medical history. She is a retired teacher. She neither smokes nor drinks alcohol and is on no medication. Her preoperative serum creatinine was 76 μmol/L. The initial surgery was uneventful and she was given cefuroxime and metronidazole as routine antibiotic prophylaxis. However, the patient developed a prolonged ileus associated with abdominal pain. On postoperative day 5, the patient started to spike fevers up to 38.5°C and was commenced on intravenous gentamicin 80 mg 8 hourly in addition to the other antibiotics. Over the next 5 days, she remained persistently febrile, with negative blood cultures. In the last 24 h, she has also become relatively hypotensive, with her systolic blood pressure around 95 mmHg despite intravenous colloids. Her urine output is now 15 mL/h.

Examination

She is unwell and sweating profusely. She is jaundiced. Her pulse rate is 110/min regular, blood pressure is 95/60 mmHg and jugular venous pressure is not raised. Her heart sounds are normal. Her respiratory rate is 30/min. Her breath sounds are normal. Her abdomen is tender, with guarding over the right iliac fossa. Bowel sounds are absent.

🔍 INVESTIGATIONS

		Normal
Haemoglobin	8.2 g/dL	11.7–15.7 g/dL
Mean corpuscular volume (MCV)	83 fL	80–99 fL
White cell count	26.3 × 10⁹/L	3.5–11.0 × 10⁹/L
Platelets	94 × 10⁹/L	150–440 × 10⁹/L
Sodium	126 mmol/L	135–145 mmol/L
Potassium	5.8 mmol/L	3.5–5.0 mmol/L
Bicarbonate	6 mmol/L	24–30 mmol/L
Urea	36.2 mmol/L	2.5–6.7 mmol/l
Creatinine	523 μmol/L	70–120 μmol/L
Glucose	2.6 mmol/L	4.0–6.0 mmol/L
Albumin	31 g/L	35–50 g/L
Bilirubin	95 mmol/L	3–17 mmol/L
Alanine transaminase	63 IU/L	5–35 IU/L
Alkaline phosphatase	363 IU/L	30–300 IU/L
Trough gentamicin level	4.8 mg/mL	<2.0 mg/mL

Urinalysis: + blood; + protein; granular casts and epithelial cells

❓ QUESTIONS

- What are the causes of this patient's acute renal failure?
- How would you further investigate this patient?
- How would you manage this patient?

DOI: 10.1201/9781003350934-81

ANSWER 73

This woman has postoperative acute renal failure due to a combination of intra-abdominal sepsis and aminoglycoside nephrotoxicity. Her sepsis is due to an anastomotic leak with local-ised peritonitis, which has been partially controlled with antibiotics. Her sepsis syndrome is manifested by fever, tachycardia, hypotension, hypoglycaemia, metabolic acidosis (low bicar-bonate) and oliguria. The low sodium and high potassium are common in this condition as cell membrane function becomes less effective. The elevated white count is a marker for bacterial infection, and the low platelet count is part of the picture of disseminated intravascular coagula-tion. Jaundice and abnormal liver function tests are common features of intra-abdominal sepsis. Aminoglycosides (gentamicin, streptomycin, amikacin) cause auditory and vestibular dysfunc-tion, as well as acute renal failure. Risk factors for aminoglycoside nephrotoxicity are higher doses and duration of treatment, increased age, pre-existing renal insufficiency, hepatic failure and volume depletion. Aminoglycoside nephrotoxicity usually occurs 7–10 days after starting treatment. Monitoring of trough levels is important, although an increase in the trough level generally indicates decreased excretion of the drug caused by a fall in the glomerular flow rate. Thus, nephrotoxicity may be already established by the time the trough level rises.

This patient needs urgent resuscitation. She requires transfer to the intensive care unit, where she will need invasive circulatory monitoring with an arterial line and central venous pressure line to allow accurate assessment of her colloid and inotrope requirements. She also needs urgent renal replacement therapy to correct her acidosis and hyperkalaemia. In a haemodynamically unstable patient like this, continuous haemofiltration is the preferred method. She also needs urgent surgical review. The abdomen should be imaged with either ultrasound or computed tomography (CT) scanning to try to identify any collection of pus. Once haemodynamically stable, the patient should have a laparotomy to drain any collection and form a temporary colostomy.

 KEY POINTS

- Postoperative acute renal failure is often multifactorial due to hypotension, sepsis and the use of nephrotoxic drugs such as aminoglycosides and non-steroidal anti-inflammatory drugs (NSAIDs).
- Aminoglycoside drugs are extremely valuable for treating gram-negative infections, but levels must be monitored to avoid toxicity.
- Sepsis syndrome must be recognised early and treated aggressively to reduce the morbidity and mortality of this condition.

CASE 74: BLOOD IN THE URINE

History

A 52-year-old businessman is referred to a nephrologist for investigation of microscopic hae-maturia. This was first detected 6 months ago at an insurance medical for a new job and has since been confirmed on two occasions by his general practitioner (GP). His blood pressure was mildly elevated as his last medical exam. Previous urinalyses have been normal. He has never had macroscopic haematuria and has no urinary symptoms. He is otherwise in excellent health. There is no significant past medical history. He has no symptoms of visual problems or deafness. There is no family history of renal disease. He drinks 35 units of alcohol per week and smokes 30 cigarettes per day.

Examination

He is a fit-looking, well-nourished man. His pulse is 72/min; blood pressure is 146/102 mmHg. Otherwise, examination of his cardiovascular, respiratory, abdominal and neurological systems is unremarkable. Fundoscopy reveals arteriovenous nipping.

🔍 INVESTIGATIONS

		Normal
Haemoglobin	13.6 g/dL	13.3–17.7 g/dL
Mean corpuscular volume (MCV)	83 fL	80–99 fL
White cell count	4.2×10^9/L	3.9–10.6×10^9/L
Platelets	213×10^9/L	150–440×10^9/L
Sodium	138 mmol/L	135–145 mmol/L
Potassium	3.8 mmol/L	3.5–5.0 mmol/L
Urea	8.2 mmol/L	2.5–6.7 mmol/L
Creatinine	141 µmol/L	70–120 µmol/L
Albumin	38 g/L	35–50 g/L
Glucose	4.5 mmol/L	4.0–6.0 mmol/L
Bilirubin	13 mmol/L	3–17 mmol/L
Alanine transaminase	33 IU/L	5–35 IU/L
Alkaline phosphatase	72 IU/L	30–300 IU/L
Gamma-glutamyl transpeptidase	211 IU/L	11–51 IU/L

Urinalysis: ++ protein; ++ blood; >100 red cells

24-h urinary protein: 1.2 g; normal <200 mg/24 h

Electrocardiogram (ECG): left ventricular hypertrophy

Renal ultrasound: two normal-size kidneys

❓ QUESTIONS

- What is the likely diagnosis?
- What further investigations would you organise?
- What advice would you give this patient?

ANSWER 74

Microscopic haematuria has many renal and urological causes (e.g., prostatic disease, stones), but the presence of significant proteinuria, hypertension and renal impairment suggest this man has some form of chronic glomerulonephritis. The high gamma-glutamyl transpeptidase level is compatible with liver disease related to his high alcohol intake. The recommended upper limit for men is 28 units per week.

> **!   COMMONEST GLOMERULAR CAUSES OF MICROSCOPIC HAEMATURIA**
>
> - Immunoglobulin A (IgA) nephropathy
> - Thin basement membrane disease
> - Alport's syndrome (predominantly affects males)

IgA nephropathy is the commonest glomerulonephritis in developed countries and is characterised by diffuse mesangial deposits of IgA immune complexes. Patients often have episodes of macroscopic haematuria concurrent with upper respiratory tract infection. Most cases of IgA nephropathy are idiopathic, but it is also commonly associated with Henoch-Schönlein purpura and alcoholic cirrhosis. This man has IgA nephropathy in association with alcoholic liver disease. About 20% of patients with IgA nephropathy will develop end-stage renal failure after 20 years of follow-up.

Thin basement membrane disease is a familial disorder that presents with isolated microscopic haematuria, minimal proteinuria and normal renal function that does not deteriorate. Electron microscopy shows diffuse thinning of the glomerular basement membranes (the width is usually 150–225 nm versus 300–400 nm in normal subjects). Alport's syndrome is a progressive form of glomerular disease associated with deafness and ocular abnormalities and is usually inherited as an X-linked dominant condition, so males are more seriously affected.

This patient should have a renal biopsy to reach a histological diagnosis. Mesangial hypercellularity, positive immunofluorescence for IgA and complement protein 3 seen in the glomerulus on histology points towards the diagnosis of IgA nephropathy. As the patient is over age 50, he should have urine cytology, prostate-specific antigen and cystoscopy performed to exclude concurrent bladder and prostatic lesions. He also needs a liver ultrasound, and liver biopsy should be considered.

The patient should be advised to abstain from alcohol and needs to have his blood pressure controlled. He needs regular follow-up as he is at risk of progressing to dialysis or renal transplantation. The raised creatinine appears modest in terms of the actual figures, but as plasma/serum creatinine does not begin to rise until the glomerular filtration rate is reduced to 50% of normal (irrespective of the patient's age), the raised creatinine in this case indicates a serious loss of renal function to approximately 40% of normal. There is no convincing evidence for immunosuppression retarding the progression into renal failure in most patients with IgA nephropathy; however, initial treatment with angiotensin-converting enzyme inhibitor may improve persistent proteinuria (>500–1000 mg/day).

> **KEY POINTS**
>
> - Patients with isolated haematuria aged older than 50 years should be initially referred to a urologist for investigation to exclude bladder or prostatic disease.
> - Small elevations in serum/plasma creatinine indicate large loss in renal function.
> - Liver damage from high alcohol intake may occur with no obvious signs and symptoms.

CASE 75: KIDNEY FAILURE

History

A 48-year-old woman is seen by her GP complaining of tiredness for several months. She also has suffered from headaches over the past 6 weeks for which she has been taking regular ibuprofen. She has no significant past medical history. She has two children aged 16 and 13. Her pregnancies were uncomplicated. She has complained of painful periods over many years for which she has taken a variety of non-steroidal anti-inflammatory drugs (NSAIDs) and over-the-counter herbal remedies.

Examination

She looks pale. Her pulse is 84/min regular, blood pressure 178/102 mmHg, jugular venous pressure not raised and heart sounds normal. Her respiratory and abdominal examinations are normal. Neurological examination is normal. Fundoscopy shows arteriovenous nipping and silver-wiring of the retinal vessels.

INVESTIGATIONS		
		Normal
Haemoglobin	12.0 g/dL	11.7–15.7 g/dL
White cell count	10.8×10^9/L	$3.5–11.0 \times 10^9$/L
Platelets	154×10^9/L	$150–440 \times 10^9$/L
Sodium	137 mmol/L	135–145 mmol/L
Potassium	4.8 mmol/L	3.5–5.0 mmol/L
Urea	12.1 mmol/L	2.5–6.7 mmol/L
Creatinine	375 µmol/L	70–120 µmol/L
Bicarbonate	18 mmol/L	24–30 mmol/L
Glucose	4.5 mmol/L	4.0–6.0 mmol/L

Urinalysis: ≤ protein; – blood

? QUESTIONS

- What are the potential causes of this patient's renal failure?
- What further investigations are indicated for this patient?
- How would you manage this patient?

DOI: 10.1201/9781003350934-83

ANSWER 75

This woman has significant renal failure with associated acidosis and anaemia. Her urinalysis is negative, which excludes a glomerular disease. It is more likely that her renal failure is due to either tubulointerstitial disease or disease affecting the renal vasculature such as accelerated phase hypertension. Potential causes of tubulointerstitial disease in this case are NSAIDs and herbal medicines. Her hypertension is likely secondary to her tubulointerstitial disease and is accelerating the progression of her renal failure.

NSAIDs cause acute kidney injury by two different mechanisms: haemodynamically mediated and acute interstitial nephritis. Haemodynamically mediated acute renal failure is due to inhibition of prostaglandin synthesis. Prostaglandins cause prerenal vasodilatation which is crucial to maintain renal perfusion in the setting of hypovolaemia, cirrhosis and heart failure. In this case, there is no evidence that she is dehydrated. NSAIDs also cause an acute interstitial nephritis. There may be an associated fever, rash, eosinophilia and eosinophiluria. Urine microscopy may show sterile pyuria and white cell casts. Histological findings from a kidney biopsy often show marked interstitial oedema and infiltrate in the connective tissue between renal tubules. Spontaneous recovery occurs within a few months after the NSAID is discontinued, although there may be permanent renal damage. A course of prednisolone is generally given to accelerate renal recovery and lessen long-term scarring. NSAIDs can also induce minimal change disease and membranous nephropathy causing nephritic syndrome. In addition to these acute effects, it has been suggested that daily NSAID use for a prolonged period may be associated with an increased risk of chronic kidney disease, although the percentage of patients is small relative to the number of NSAIDs that are bought over the counter.

In this case, it is important to find out if her renal failure is acute or long-standing. This can easily be discovered if she has had previous measurements of her serum creatinine. Renal ultrasound is also helpful. If the ultrasound shows small echogenic kidneys, her renal failure is likely chronic. If her kidneys are normal in size, a renal biopsy is indicated to confirm the diagnosis and assess the extent of inflammation and scarring.

In this case, her renal failure is likely due to a NSAID-induced interstitial nephritis. She should be advised to stop her NSAIDs and herbal medicines, and never to restart these drugs. She should be given a short course of prednisolone to hasten renal recovery.

 KEY POINTS

- A full drug history is vital in patients with unexplained renal failure.
- NSAIDs are the most common drug implicated in acute interstitial nephritis.
- Aristolochic acid-containing herbal medicines cause a characteristic nephropathy.

Section 9

INFECTIOUS DISEASES AND MICROBIOLOGY

History

A 24-year-old man presents to his general practitioner (GP) with 3 days of intermittent fever. He complains of feeling cold and shivery and at other times very sweaty, he has progressively become exhausted and unwell.

There is a history of hepatitis 4 years earlier, and glandular fever at the age of 18. He smokes 15–20 cigarettes each day and occasionally smokes marijuana. He denies any intravenous drug abuse. He drinks about 14 units of alcohol each week. He is heterosexual and has had a number of recent sexual partners, all with condoms. He returned from Nigeria 3 weeks ago and has almost completed his anti-malarial prophylaxis. He was in Nigeria for 6 weeks working for an oil company and reports he was well there.

Examination

He looks unwell. His pulse is 94/min, blood pressure is 118/72 mmHg and temperature is 38.7°C. Cardiac and respiratory examination is normal. In the abdomen, there is some tenderness in the left upper quadrant. There are no enlarged lymph nodes.

🔍 INVESTIGATIONS

		Normal
Haemoglobin	11.1 g/dL	13.7–17.7 g/dL
Mean corpuscular volume (MCV)	97 fL	80–99 fL
White cell count	9.4×10^9/L	$3.9–10.6 \times 10^9$/L
Neutrophils	6.3×10^9/L	$1.8–7.7 \times 10^9$/L
Lymphocytes	2.9×10^9/L	$1.0–4.8 \times 10^9$/L
Platelets	88×10^9/L	$150–440 \times 10^9$/L
Sodium	134 mmol/L	135–145 mmol/L
Potassium	4.8 mmol/L	3.5–5.0 mmol/L
Urea	4.2 mmol/L	2.5–6.7 mmol/L
Creatinine	74 µmol/L	70 120 µmol/L
Alkaline phosphatase	76 IU/L	30–300 IU/L
Alanine aminotransferase	33 IU/L	5–35 IU/L
Gamma-glutamyl transpeptidase	42 IU/L	11–51 IU/L
Bilirubin	28 mmol/L	3–17 mmol/L
Glucose	4.5 mmol/L	4.0–6.0 mmol/L

Urine: no protein, no blood, no sugar
Blood cultures pending.

❓ QUESTIONS

- What is the most likely diagnosis?
- What abnormalities are likely to be present in the blood film?
- What would be the appropriate management?

ANSWER 76

The most important features in this 24-year-old are the fever and rigors. He looks unwell, with tachycardia and tenderness in the left upper quadrant potentially related to splenic enlargement.

There is a raised bilirubin with normal liver enzymes, anaemia of 11.1 g/dL with a normal mean corpuscular volume and a low platelet count. This makes haemolytic anaemia likely. Recent travel to Nigeria raises the suspicion of malaria. The incubation period depends on the malarial species, but can be anywhere from 7 to 30 days, with *Plasmodium falciparum* often having a shorter incubation period. Longer incubation periods occur in semi-immune individuals (e.g., people who live in endemic areas) and persons taking inadequate malaria prophylaxis. The haemolytic anaemia with a low platelet count are typical findings and relate to haemolysis during the malarial lifecycle. Splenomegaly may occur due to the spleen filtering infected red cells.

The diagnosis should be confirmed by expert examination of a Giemsa or Wright's-stained blood film with thick and thin smears, which, in this case, showed parasitised red blood cells demonstrated by the classic ring-shaped trophozoites of *P. falciparum* inside the red blood cells. The degree of parasitaemia can also be estimated from a blood film (1% in this case).

Malaria prophylaxis is often not adhered to very well. Even when taken as advised, it does not offer complete protection. A thorough travel history, including history of vaccination, exposures and insect bites should be obtained.

His history does not suggest particular risk factors for human immunodeficiency virus (HIV) infection (such as intravenous drug abuse or high-risk sexual behaviours), although it is difficult to rule out on history alone. HIV seroconversion can produce a feverish illness, but usually not as severe as this case. Nevertheless, an HIV test should be performed. Blood cultures must always be collected in fever in a returning traveller. Other acute arboviral infections such as dengue or bacterial infections such as rickettsia are differentials for his clinical presentation.

Treatment depends on local resistance patterns, and up-to-date advice should be sought from microbiology or tropical disease specialists. *Falciparum* malaria is usually treated with artemisinin derivatives such as artesunate IV or oral drugs such as Riamet, depending on the severity. In severe cases, hyponatraemia and hypoglycaemia may occur. Most of the severe complications are associated with *P. falciparum* malaria as opposed to other species.

 SIGNS AND SYMPTOMS OF SEVERE MALARIA

- Cerebral malaria
- Acute respiratory distress syndrome
- Severe haemolysis
- Acute renal failure

In *Plasmodium vivax* or *Plasmodium ovale* infection, the patient may have hypnozoites – a dormant form of the parasite which can remain in the liver and activate at a later stage resulting in disease relapse. Hypnozoite eradication can be achieved by prescribing primaquine (this is usually given after the patient has recovered from acute infection). Patients who are given primaquine need to have their glucose-6-phosphate dehydrogenase (G6PD) levels checked as primaquine can cause severe haemolysis in patients with G6PD deficiency.

Another important aspect of management is patient education on bite avoidance, such as using repellent or insect nets, and ensuring up-to-date travel vaccinations for other infectious diseases.

 KEY POINTS

- No prophylactic regime is certain to prevent malaria.
- Malaria is one of the most common causes of fever in returning traveller, and anyone returning from an endemic area with fever must have a malarial blood film requested.
- Treatment should be guided by advice from local microbiology departments. Complex cases can be discussed with tropical disease centres.
- If the malaria species is unknown or the infection mixed, treat as *falciparum* malaria, as this causes the most severe disease.

CASE 77: FEVERS AND MALAISE

History

A 54-year-old woman attends the emergency department with a 5-day history of fever and malaise. She also reports a non-productive cough.

Her past medical history includes hypertension and insulin-dependent diabetes. She received a deceased donor renal transplant 18 months ago for deteriorating renal function. Three episodes of rejection have been treated with increasing doses of immunosuppression. She had been taking co-trimoxazole prophylaxis but this was discontinued at 12 months post-transplant.

Examination

On examination, her temperature is 38°C, blood pressure 132/82, pulse 86/min, respiratory rate 20/min and oxygen saturation 94%. No abnormalities are found in the cardiovascular or respiratory system. There is no tenderness over the transplanted kidney and no lymphadenopathy.

🔍 INVESTIGATIONS

		Normal
Haemoglobin	12.8 g/dL	13.3–17.7 g/dL
Mean corpuscular volume (MCV)	89 fL	80–99 fL
White cell count	8.2×10^9/L	$3.9–10.6 \times 10^9$/L
Neutrophils	7.6×10^9/L	$1.8–7.7 \times 10^9$/L
Lymphocytes	0.2×10^9/L	$0.6–4.8 \times 10^9$/L
Monocytes	0.2×10^9/L	$0.6–1.0 \times 10^9$/L
Platelets	221×10^9/L	$150–440 \times 10^9$/L
Sodium	134 mmol/L	135–145 mmol/L
Potassium	4.3 mmol/L	3.5–5.0 mmol/L
Urea	7.2 mmol/L	2.5–6.7 mmol/L
Creatinine	141 µmol/L	70–120 µmol/L
Bilirubin	16 mmol/L	3–17 mmol/L
Alanine transaminase	29 IU/L	5–35 IU/L
Gamma-glutamyl transaminase	53 IU/L	11–51 IU/L
Alkaline phosphatase	251 IU/L	30–300 IU/L
LDH	450 IU/L	14–280 IU/L

Urinalysis: no protein; no blood

Chest radiograph: normal

She is treated with paracetamol and asked to return if there was any deterioration. Three days later, she returns with more frequent fever, ongoing cough and a new problem of shortness of breath. On examination, her temperature is now 38.8°C, blood pressure 122/78, pulse 90/min, respiratory rate 26/min and oxygen saturation 92%.

❓ QUESTIONS

- What is the most likely diagnosis?
- What further investigations are indicated for this patient?
- How would you manage this patient?

ANSWER 77

Fever in transplant patients is often caused by common pathogens, but immunosuppression raises the possibility of an opportunistic infection. The possibility is higher here because of the increased immunosuppression secondary to the episodes of rejection.

The symptoms of dry cough and shortness of breath point to a respiratory focus. Although lung auscultation is normal and the chest radiograph is clear, tachypnoea is present and the decrease in oxygen saturation confirms a significant problem with gas exchange in the lung.

The combination of a fever, dry cough with no respiratory signs and worsening hypoxia in an immunosuppressed patient is suggestive of *Pneumocystis jirovecii* pneumonia, a fungal pneumonia. The chest radiograph may appear normal in the early stages before diffuse shadowing develops, with an alveolar filling pattern most marked in the mid- and lower zones, often sparing the costophrenic angles (Figure 77.1). This patient was taking co-trimoxazole as prophylaxis against *Pneumocystis* but this was stopped because of a rash, increasing the risk of infection.

The first investigation here should be a chest radiograph. Even if expectorating, *P. jirovecii* is not easily identified in the sputum and usually requires bronchoscopy with alveolar lavage to sample deeper alveolar contents. *P. jirovecii* is a fungus which is found in the environment and usually causes infection in those who are significantly immunosuppressed. Samples from alveolar lavage are stained with a silver stain, periodic acid Schiff or immunofluorescence. Polymerase chain reaction (PCR) to detect *P. jirovecii* DNA can also be performed. PCR is highly sensitive and specific for detecting *Pneumocystis*; however, it cannot distinguish colonisation from disease, although higher organism loads as determined by quantitative PCR (Q-PCR) assays are likely to represent clinically significant disease. A component of the cell wall of fungi, 1,3 β-D-glucan (Beta-D-Glucan) can also aid diagnosis and is often elevated in the blood of patients with pneumocystis pneumonia.

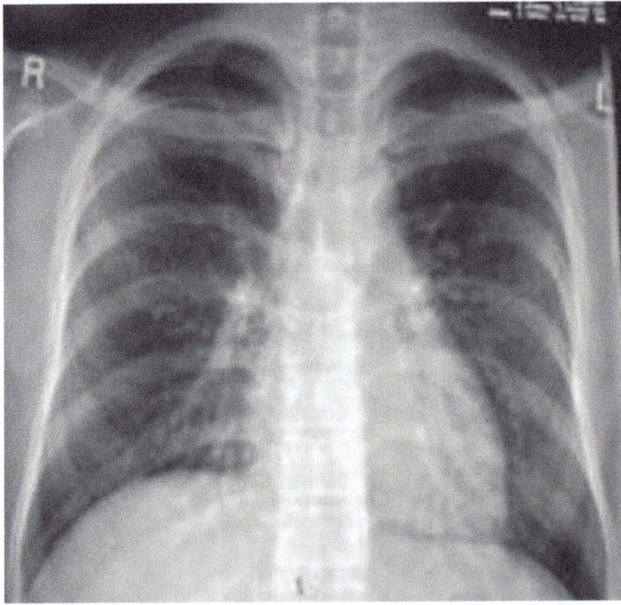

Figure 77.1 Chest radiograph.

Treatment is with high-dose co-trimoxazole with steroids depending on oxygen saturations (p_aO_2 <7.3 is the cut off for starting high-dose steroids). The previous rash to co-trimoxazole means that alternative treatments such as dapsone and trimethoprim or clindamycin and primaquine may be used. This should be done in conjunction with microbiology or infectious diseases teams.

🔑 KEY POINTS

- *Pneumocystis jirovecii* is a ubiquitous fungus which can cause disease in immunosuppressed patients.
- Dry cough, fever and breathlessness are common symptoms with tachypnoea and significant hypoxia.
- Diagnosis usually requires sampling of alveolar contents by lavage.
- Treatment involves steroids and co-trimoxazole.

CASE 78: SHORTNESS OF BREATH ON EXERTION

History

A 23-year-old student presents to her general practitioner (GP) complaining of shortness of breath on exertion. This has developed over the past 10 days, and she is now breathless after walking 50 yards. About 2 weeks ago, she had a flu-like illness with generalised muscle aches and fever. She feels extremely tired and has noticed palpitations in association with her breathlessness. In addition, she has some discomfort in her chest that is worse on inspiration. Previously, she has been extremely fit with no significant past medical history. There is no recent history of foreign travel. She denies substance abuse.

Examination

On examination, her temperature is 37.5°C. Her pulse rate is 120/min and regular. Blood pressure is 90/70 mmHg. Jugular venous pressure is raised at 8 cm. On auscultation, there is a gallop rhythm with a third heart sound. Examination of her chest is unremarkable. Pressure over the sternum causes discomfort. Abdominal and neurological examinations are normal.

🔍 INVESTIGATIONS

The GP sends the student to the emergency department, where an electrocardiogram (ECG) and chest radiograph are performed. The ECG shows T-wave flattening globally. The chest radiograph is shown in Figure 78.1.

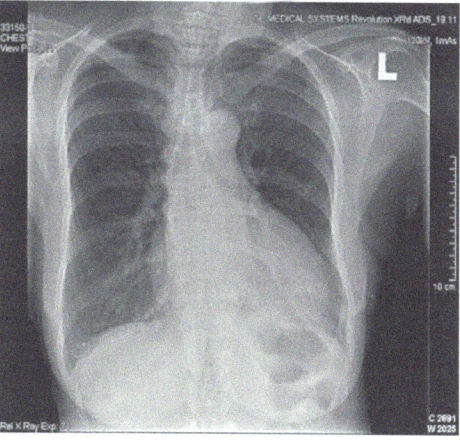

Figure 78.1 Chest radiograph.

❓ QUESTIONS

- What is the likely diagnosis?
- How would you further investigate?
- How would you manage this patient?

DOI: 10.1201/9781003350934-87

ANSWER 78

This patient has viral myocarditis, likely due to Coxsackie B virus. Viruses that can cause myocarditis include Coxsackie B and A, echovirus, adenovirus, influenza, varicella, polio, mumps, rabies, viral hepatitis, rubella, parvovirus B19, Epstein-Barr virus (EBV), cytomegalovirus (CMV) and herpes simplex virus. Myocarditis also may occur during bacteraemia or fungaemia. *Rickettsia* and diphtheria can cause myocarditis. In rural South America, acute infection with the protozoan Trypanosoma cruzi causes fever, myocarditis and hepatosplenomegaly, and 10–30 years later, this can lead to cardiac failure and conduction system defects (Chagas disease). Cocaine abuse can cause myocarditis and sudden death. Profound hypocalcaemia, hypophosphataemia and hypomagnesaemia can all cause myocardial depression.

The clinical picture of myocarditis is non-specific, but common symptoms include myalgia, fatigue, shortness of breath, pericardial pain and palpitations. Myocarditis should be suspected in a young person presenting with new onset cardiac symptoms. There is often a prodromal viral illness affecting the upper respiratory tract or gastrointestinal system. Autoimmune diseases such as lupus should be excluded, and a careful social history should be taken to exclude alcohol or cocaine abuse. The main clinical signs are those of cardiac failure. A pericardial friction rub may be heard in some patients with myopericarditis. Patients usually have a marked sinus tachycardia disproportionate to the slight fever. ECG usually shows ST segment and T-wave abnormalities. There may be atrial or, more commonly, ventricular arrhythmias or signs of conducting system defects. The chest radiograph may be normal if the myocarditis is mild, but if there is cardiac failure, there will be cardiomegaly and pulmonary congestion. The differential diagnoses in this case include hypertrophic cardiomyopathy, pericarditis and myocardial ischaemia.

Cardiac enzymes such as troponin I or T and creatine kinase are raised. Echocardiography should be performed to confirm the diagnosis. Echocardiographic changes may be focal affecting only the right or left ventricle, or global. There is poor contractility of the myocardium. Cardiac enzymes such as troponin I or T and creatine kinase are raised. Cardiac magnetic resonance imaging can detect myocardial oedema and myocyte injury in myocarditis. Coronary angiography may be performed to exclude coronary artery disease. Endomyocardial biopsy is considered depending on the course and severity of the condition. Paired serum samples should be taken for antibody titres to Coxsackie B and mumps.

Bed rest is the treatment for the period of acute viral myocarditis. Diuretics and angiotensin-converting enzyme (ACE) inhibitors are used to treat cardiac failure. Anticoagulation may be required for patients with intracardiac thrombi. There is controversy over treatment with corticosteroids; they tend to be used in patients with a short history, a positive endomyocardial biopsy, and the most severe cases. Most cases are benign and self-limiting, and cardiac function will return to normal. However, a minority will develop permanent cardiac damage, leading to dilated cardiomyopathy. Definitive treatment may then involve cardiac transplantation.

🔑 **KEY POINTS**

- The features in favour of the diagnosis of viral myocarditis include the young age of the patient, the preceding acute febrile illness and, subsequently, the raised serum antibody titres to Coxsackie B.
- It is important to take a history of foreign travel, alcohol intake and substance abuse.
- Outcome in adults is generally good, but a proportion of patients will develop dilated cardiomyopathy.

CASE 79: HEADACHES AND CONFUSION

History

A 28-year-old Ghanian nurse is admitted to the emergency department complaining of headaches and confusion. Her headaches developed over the past 3 weeks and have progressively worsened, becoming persistent and diffuse. Her friend who accompanies her says that she has lost 10 kg in weight over 6 months and has recently become disoriented and confused. While in the emergency department, she has a generalised tonic-clonic convulsion which self-terminates after 1 minute.

Examination

She is thin and weighs 55 kg. Her temperature is 38.5°C. There is oral candidiasis. There is cervical lymphadenopathy. Examination of her cardiovascular, respiratory and gastrointestinal systems is normal. She is disoriented in time, place and person. There were no focal neurological signs. Fundoscopy shows bilateral papilloedema.

🔍 INVESTIGATIONS

		Normal
Haemoglobin	12.2 g/dL	11.7–15.7 g/dL
White cell count	12.1 × 10⁹/L	3.5–11.0 × 10⁹/L
Lymphocytes	0.6 × 10⁹/L	1.0-4.0 × 10⁹/L
Platelets	131 × 10⁹/L	150–440 × 10⁹/L
Sodium	126 mmol/L	135–145 mmol/L
Potassium	3.9 mmol/L	3.5–5.0 mmol/L
Urea	6.2 mmol/L	2.5–6.7 mmol/L
Creatinine	73 μmol/L	70–120 μmol/L
Glucose	5.6 mmol/L	4.0–6.0 mmol/L

A computed tomography (CT) scan is shown in Figure 79.1.

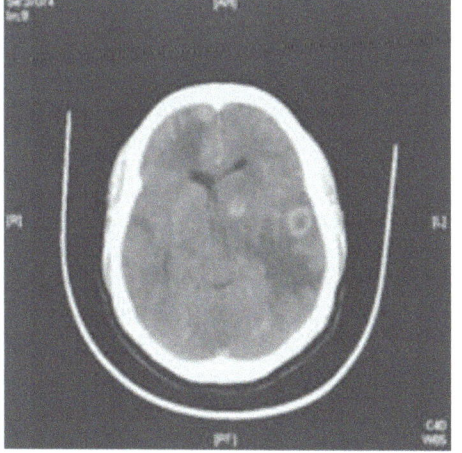

Figure 79.1 Computed tomography scan of the brain.

❓ QUESTIONS

- What is the cause for this woman's headaches, confusion and convulsions?
- What is the underlying diagnosis?
- How should this woman be further investigated and treated?

DOI: 10.1201/9781003350934-88

ANSWER 79

This woman has cerebral toxoplasmosis secondary to human immunodeficiency virus (HIV) infection. This condition is caused by the protozoan *Toxoplasma gondii*, which primarily infects cats but can be carried by any warm-blooded animal. Human infection most commonly occurs by ingesting food or water contaminated by cat faeces or by eating raw meat containing *Toxoplasma* cysts. After ingestion the organism spreads to muscles and the brain. The immune system rapidly controls the infection and the cysts become dormant (latent infection).

The primary infection is generally asymptomatic but can cause an acute mononucleosis-type illness with generalised lymphadenopathy and rash. It may leave scars in the choroid and retina and small inflammatory lesions in the brain.

If the patient becomes immunocompromised, the infection reactivates, causing toxoplasmosis. This is a common condition in people with advanced HIV and acquired immune deficiency syndrome (AIDS) but is relatively rare in solid-organ transplant recipients.

Cerebral toxoplasmosis usually presents with a subacute illness comprising fever, headache, confusion, convulsions, cognitive disturbance and focal neurological signs, including hemiparesis, ataxia, cranial nerve lesions, visual field defects and sensory loss. Movement disorders are common due to involvement of the basal ganglia. Computed tomography (CT) or magnetic resonance imaging will usually show multiple bilateral ring-enhancing lesions, predominantly located near the grey-white matter junction, basal ganglia, brainstem and cerebellum.

The clinical and radiological differential diagnoses include lymphoma, tuberculosis, *Cryptococcus*, syphilitic gumma, metastases and bacterial abscesses. Anti-toxoplasma immunoglobulin G (IgG) antibody is usually positive in patients with cerebral toxoplasmosis, and toxoplasma polymerase chain reaction (PCR) can be performed on cerebrospinal fluid.

The headaches and papilloedema are caused by raised intracranial pressure from the multiple space-occupying lesions. The hyponatraemia is due to the syndrome of inappropriate antidiuretic hormone secretion consequent to the raised intracranial pressure.

This woman should be started on anticonvulsants to prevent further seizures. Treatment is started with high-dose sulfadiazine and pyrimethamine together with folinic acid to prevent myelosuppression (a potential side-effect of the treatment). There should be a clinical and radiological improvement by 2 weeks. If there is no improvement, a biopsy of one of the lesions should be considered. Cerebral toxoplasmosis is uniformly fatal if untreated and, even with treatment, neurological complications may occur.

Clues for HIV infection include weight loss, oral candidiasis and lymphadenopathy. An HIV test should be obtained, alongside a CD4 count. She should be referred to sexual health or infectious diseases for ongoing follow-up of her HIV with a view to initiating antiretrovirals once her toxoplasma has been adequately treated. Partner notification is important so previous/current partners have the opportunity to get tested. The patient can do this herself or the sexual health department can do this anonymously on her behalf. She should be encouraged to inform her occupational health team; however, unless she is performing exposure-prone procedures, risk of transmission to patients is negligible.

🔑 KEY POINTS

- Toxoplasmosis is the most common opportunistic infection of the central nervous system in patients with AIDS.
- Patients can present with headache, confusion, seizures and focal neurological deficits.
- The clinical and radiological response to treatment should be observed by 2 weeks. No improvement by this time should prompt re-evaluation and further investigation.

CASE 80: CONFUSION

History

A 79-year-old man has lived in a residential home for 3 years since his wife died. He was unable to look after himself at home because osteoarthritis of his hips limited his mobility. Otherwise, apart from a rather irritable temper, he has had no problems in residential care.

However, he has become more difficult in the last 36 h. He has accused staff of assaulting him and stealing his money. He has gotten out of bed unaided, resulting in a fall. He has become incontinent of urine over the last 24 h, which is not usual for him. The duty doctor reviews and finds he is rather sleepy. When roused, he seems frightened and becomes verbally aggressive. He thinks the staff are having secret meetings and planning to harm him. When questioned, he doesn't know where he is or the time or date.

He is a non-smoker and drinks 1–2 units of alcohol a month. On a routine blood test 8 years ago, he was diagnosed with hypothyroidism and thyroxine 100 mg daily is the only medication he is taking regularly. His records show his thyroid function was normal 6 months ago.

The nursing staff say he is now too difficult to manage in the residential home. They feel he has dementia, and that the home is not an appropriate place for such patients.

Examination

Confusion and disorientation are noted. Blood pressure is 178/102 mmHg. Bilateral hip movement is limited due to pain. His abdomen is soft though the suprapubic area is tender on palpation. He has been incontinent of urine.

🔍 INVESTIGATIONS

		Normal
Thyroxine	125 nmol/L	70–140 nmol/L
Thyroid-stimulating hormone	1.6 mU/L	0.3–6.0 mU/L
Blood glucose	6.2 mmol/L	4.0–6.0 mmol/L

C-reactive protein (CRP) 45

Urine dipstick: – sugar, + protein, ++ blood, leucocytes +++, nitrites positive

---

❓ QUESTIONS

- What is the likely diagnosis?
- What investigations are indicated?
- How should the patient be managed?

DOI: 10.1201/9781003350934-89

ANSWER 80

This case demonstrates delirium. The four key features that characterise delirium are disturbance of consciousness, no obvious pre-existing dementia, confusion that develops acutely (over hours or days) and tends to fluctuate during the day. In contrast, the cognitive changes in dementia are insidious, progressive and occur over a longer time frame.

Delirium is caused by an inciting event such as fluid and electrolyte disturbances, infections, drug or alcohol toxicity or withdrawal, metabolic disorders (hypoglycaemia, hypercalcaemia, liver failure), low perfusion states (shock, heart failure) and postoperative states.

In this case, there is no record of any drugs except thyroxine, although this should be rechecked to rule out analgesics or other agents that he might have had recently prescribed. The lack of thyroid replacement for 2 days will not have a significant effect and the normal results 6 months earlier make this an unlikely cause of his delirium.

His glucose is normal. The falls raise the possibility of trauma, and a subdural haematoma could present in this way. However, it seems that the falls were a secondary phenomenon. The most likely cause is that he has a urinary tract infection (UTI). There is blood, protein, leucocytes and nitrites on his urine dipstick, he has become incontinent and he has some suprapubic tenderness, which could fit with a lower UTI. Even simple UTIs can precipitate delirium in the elderly.

Simple UTIs can be treated with oral antibiotics in the community. Avoiding hospital admission would be beneficial for this patient because moving to a new environment can worsen delirium. Delirium generally improves once the precipitant has been resolved or treated, but it may persist for some time even after physical symptoms such as fever have settled.

Urine should be sent for microscopy, culture and sensitivity, and empirical treatment for UTI can be started in accordance with local microbiology guidance. The most likely organism is *Escherichia coli*, and an antibiotic such as trimethoprim or nitrofurantoin is usually first-line. The confusion should be treated calmly, consistently and without confrontation. If medication is necessary, small doses of a neuroleptic such as haloperidol or olanzapine may help, and this can be discussed with psychiatry and/or care of the elderly teams.

 KEY POINTS

- Acute changes in mental state need to be explained even in the elderly with baseline mental problems.
- In delirium, consciousness is clouded, disorientation is usual, and delusions may develop. The onset is acute. In dementia, there is an acquired global impairment of intellect, memory and personality, but consciousness is typically clear.
- Common triggers include metabolic, pharmacological and infective insults.

History

A 36-year-old man presents to his general practitioner (GP) complaining of fever and generalised aching in his back and legs. He initially thought he had the flu, but the symptoms persisted for 10 days. He also developed a sore mouth and throat, which made it difficult to eat. At symptom onset, he noticed a mild erythematous rash over his chest and abdomen, but this has since faded.

He has attended the practice previously for travel vaccinations for Vietnam and Thailand. His last trip abroad was 3 months ago. He smokes 10 cigarettes daily, drinks 20–30 units of alcohol weekly and takes no illicit drugs. He has no other medical or family history. He works as a solicitor. He is bisexual and has had relationships with multiple men and women in the past year. Twelve months ago, he had a human immunodeficiency virus (HIV) test, which was negative.

Examination

He has a temperature of 38°C. Pulse rate is 94/min, respiratory rate is 16/min and blood pressure is 124/78 mmHg. There are no abnormalities in the cardiovascular or respiratory system. On examination of the mouth, there are two ulcers in the oral mucosa that are 5–10 mm in diameter. His pharynx is erythematous. There are a number of palpable cervical lymph nodes on both sides of the neck, which are a little tender. There are no other nodes and no enlargement of liver or spleen. There are no rashes on the skin.

🔍 INVESTIGATIONS

		Normal
Haemoglobin	14.8 g/dL	13.7–17.7 g/dL
Mean corpuscular volume (MCV)	87 fL	80–99 fL
White cell count	7.4×10^9/L	$3.9–10.6 \times 10^9$/L
Neutrophils	5.1×10^9/L	$1.8–7.7 \times 10^9$/L
Lymphocytes	$0.2.0 \times 10^9$/L	$0.6–4.8 \times 10^9$/L
Platelets	126×10^9/L	$150–440 \times 10^9$/L
Sodium	144 mmol/L	135–145 mmol/L
Potassium	4.4 mmol/L	3.5–5.0 mmol/L
Urea	5.9 mmol/L	2.5–6.7 mmol/L
Creatinine	73 µmol/L	70–120 µmol/L
Bilirubin	13 mmol/L	3–17 mmol/L
Alkaline phosphatase	121 IU/L	30–300 IU/L
Alanine aminotransferase	25 IU/L	5–35 IU/L
C-reactive protein (CRP)	36 mg/L	

Screening test for glandular fever: negative

? QUESTIONS

- What are some differential diagnoses?
- What is the most likely diagnosis?
- What is the treatment?

DOI: 10.1201/9781003350934-90

ANSWER 81

This case represents an infection with a particularly long duration of symptoms, making common respiratory viruses, such as influenza, unlikely. Other notable features are fever, rash, cervical lymphadenopathy and oral ulceration. The blood results suggest a viral infection with lymphopaenia and thrombocytopaenia. Infectious mononucleosis (glandular fever) is unlikely as this commonly causes lymphocytosis, not lymphopaenia.

The sexual history raises suspicion for sexually transmitted infections. It is possible that travel to Vietnam and Thailand may have been associated with high-risk sexual exposure. He had a negative HIV test 12 months ago. However, it is quite possible that he contracted HIV more recently and thus may now present with HIV seroconversion.

In at least 50% of cases, a seroconversion illness occurs within 4–6 weeks of acquisition. Although the HIV antibody test may be negative, this can be diagnosed by finding the presence of the HIV virus or its p24 antigen in the blood. Fourth-generation HIV tests look for both HIV antibodies and the p24 antigen. Ideally, he should have been educated on measures to reduce the risk of transmission at the time of the HIV testing 12 months prior.

This picture might also fit for secondary syphilis, which occurs 6–8 weeks after the primary lesion (chancre). However, in that case, the rash would often be more extensive, and the lymph nodes are not usually tender. A serological test for syphilis should be performed, alongside a full sexually transmitted infection screen looking for chlamydia, gonorrhoea and other blood-borne viruses. Other viral illnesses are possible. Hepatitis may present with this general prodrome, but the normal liver function tests make this unlikely. Lymphoma can present with lymphadenopathy and fever, but the oral ulceration and the rash are not typical. If the serological tests proved negative, lymph node biopsy might be considered for further diagnostics.

In this case, HIV viraemia was detected. Antiretroviral treatment should be started under the care of a sexual health or infectious diseases doctor.

 KEY POINTS

- A seroconversion illness occurs in at least 50% of people with newly acquired HIV infection and may even occur in up to 80–90%. The severity varies.
- Symptoms vary but classically consist of flu-like illness, pharyngitis, rash and lymphadenopathy. Duration may be prolonged, sometimes up to 2 weeks or longer.
- In cases of known or high-risk exposure, such as unprotected sexual intercourse with an HIV-infected person not taking antiretroviral medicine, an immediate course of antiretroviral treatment is often indicated. Immediate advice should be sought.

CASE 82: BACK PAIN

History

A 64-year-old woman presents to the hospital with 2 weeks of pain in her upper back. It radiates to her left shoulder. Additionally, she describes drenching night sweats over the previous 2 weeks and episodes of shivering. She initially managed it with over-the-counter analgesia, but the pain continued and now wakes her at night. She denies having had a fall nor any trauma. There is no recent travel and is otherwise well.

Examination

She appears well but has a temperature of 39.2°C. On examination, mild weakness is noted in her right upper limb, along with pain at the C6 level in her back. There is no lymphadenopathy and the rest of the examination is normal.

🔍 INVESTIGATIONS

		Normal
Haemoglobin	13.8 g/dL	13.3–17.7 g/dL
White cell count	15.8 × 10⁹/L	3.9–10.6 × 10⁹/L
Platelets	334 × 10⁹/L	150–440 × 10⁹/L
C-reactive protein (CRP)	150 mg/L	<5 mg/L

? QUESTIONS

- What are the differential diagnoses?
- How could you go about investigating this patient?
- What is the management?

ANSWER 82

This woman presents with subacute cervical back pain, fever and sweats. She displays red-flag symptoms such as neurological compromise, fever and pain affecting sleep. These symptoms point to a potential spinal issue. The differentials include: spinal infection (e.g., discitis osteomyelitis), spinal, disc prolapse, neoplastic processes (primary or metastases), inflammatory spondyloarthropathies and spinal fractures. The absence of trauma makes fracture or injury less likely.

The presence of fever, night sweats, along with an elevated white cell count and CRP, raises the possibility of an infection. To investigate, the first step is to ensure multiple blood cultures (ideally a minimum of 3 at different intervals) are taken to identify the responsible organism. *Staphylococcus aureus* is the most common cause of discitis when an organism is identified; other pathogens such as gram-negative enteric bacteria e.g., *Escherichia coli*, *Streptococcus pneumoniae* and *Salmonella* spp. are also common. While tuberculosis (TB) can cause discitis, its symptoms typically persist for a longer duration, often accompanied by night sweats and weight loss.

Targeted therapy can then be administered involving up to 6 weeks of antibiotics (usually at least 2 weeks intravenous followed by oral) once the causative organism is identified. Without an organism identified, empiric therapy is used but may not be as effective and there may be treatment failure. Imaging is crucial, and magnetic resonance imaging (MRI) is the gold standard. In this case, the MRI revealed discitis. Additionally, a chest radiograph (CXR) should be performed to rule out any evidence of TB. If the blood cultures do not yield positive results, the infectious disease/microbiology team should be consulted. A disc biopsy is crucial to finding the culprit pathogen and should ideally be done off antibiotics. If the patient is stable, it is appropriate to withhold antibiotics until a definitive microbiological diagnosis is made, given how important this is for definitive antibiotic treatment. In cases where the patient is not stable, a broad-spectrum antibiotic covering the aforementioned bacteria such as IV ceftriaxone may be used.

In this case, the patient had methicillin-sensitive *S. aureus* (MSSA) in her blood cultures. MSSA, a gram-positive bacterium, is typically found on the skin, but if it enters the bloodstream, for example if it breaches the skin during cellulitis, it can be highly pathogenic. MSSA has the potential to settle in specific areas. Common sites include endocarditis, discitis, abscesses and osteomyelitis. Therefore, patients with MSSA often undergo echocardiograms and focused examinations of the bones, joints and heart.

Typically, treatment involves a beta-lactam antibiotic such as flucloxacillin or cefazolin. In the case of methicillin-resistant *S. aureus* (MRSA), these antibiotics mentioned earlier are ineffective, and treatment usually requires a glycopeptide such as vancomycin or teicoplanin.

 KEY POINTS

- Blood cultures should be done before administering antibiotics in patients with fever and back pain.
- When querying discitis, an attempt should be made for spinal biopsy via orthopaedics or neurosurgical teams.
- *S. aureus* is the most common bacterial cause of discitis.
- *S. aureus* can be a normal skin commensal but is pathogenic if found in blood.
- In MSSA bacteraemia (blood-stream infection), it is vital to look for the source of infection via a structured and careful examination and investigations such as echocardiogram.
- Discitis may require prolonged treatment with antibiotics and needs a multidisciplinary (MDT) approach with microbiology/infectious disease and spinal teams.

History

A 32-year-old woman presents to hospital with severe retro-orbital headache, fever, myalgia and a blanching rash all over her body. She also complains of widespread joint pains. She recently returned from Brazil where she had been visiting friends and family. Interestingly, she mentioned her uncle had similar symptoms a few days prior in Brazil.

Examination

She looks tired, has a blanching rash and has joint and muscle pains but otherwise, the rest of her examination is normal.

🔍 INVESTIGATIONS

		Normal
Haemoglobin	13.8 g/dL	13.3–17.7 g/dL
White cell count	4.8×10^9/L	3.9–10.6×10^9/L
Platelets	70×10^9/L	150–440×10^9/L
ALT	80 IU/L	<10–50 IU/L
C-reactive protein (CRP)	150 mg/L	<5 mg/L

? QUESTIONS

- What are your differentials in this patient?
- What investigations are indicated?
- How would you manage this patient?

ANSWER 83

This woman is a febrile returning traveller. The differentials for this case include arboviruses such as the dengue, chikungunya and Zika viruses. While malaria should be considered, rashes are atypical of malaria. Given her uncle's recent infection with similar symptoms, this suggests a possible outbreak which would be more common in the arboviruses.

Other diagnoses to consider are non-tropical illnesses such as Epstein-Barr virus, cytomegalovirus, hepatitis, meningitis, syphilis, leptospirosis or human immunodeficiency virus (HIV) seroconversion. Consideration should be made for non-infective causes of rash and fever. A travel history must be obtained including a full itinerary and potential exposures (e.g., sexual, animal, insect, unwell contacts and outdoor activities).

The history of severe retro-orbital headache, blanching rash and slightly deranged liver function with low platelets are typical of an arboviral illness. This woman had dengue, a Flavivirus transmitted by the *Aedes* mosquito. Dengue is caused by one of four serologically related but distinct viruses. Most cases of severe disease occur after a second infection with a different serotype from the first.

Dengue is diagnosed with serology, e.g., immunoglobulin M (IgM) (present after about 4 days) and immunoglobulin G (IgG) or via blood polymerase chain reaction (PCR). Zika and chikungunya can be clinically indistinguishable to dengue. However, Zika virus is associated with microcephaly in neonates, and chikungunya can cause severe arthritis.

The World Health Organization (WHO) classifies dengue into three groups based on disease severity. Important markers are the platelet count, which may drop significantly, and a rising haematocrit (>20%) which is suggestive of plasma leakage. Management of dengue is supportive with fluids, analgesia transfusion and intensive care unit (ICU) support as required. Patients travelling to endemic areas should be given bite avoidance advice such as wearing long sleeves and mosquito repellent.

!   WHO 2009 CLASSIFICATION OF DENGUE

Dengue without warning signs:
- A presumptive diagnosis of dengue infection may be made in the setting of residence in or travel to an endemic area plus fever and two of the following: nausea and vomiting, rash, headache/eye pain/muscle ache or joint pain, leukopenia, positive tourniquet test (a marker of capillary fragility).

Dengue with warning signs (including above and below):
- Abdominal tenderness, persistent vomiting, clinical fluid accumulation, mucosal bleeding, lethargy or restlessness, hepatomegaly >2 cm, increase in haematocrit concentration with rapid decrease in platelets.

Severe dengue:
- Severe plasma leakage leading to:
  - Shock, fluid accumulation with respiratory distress.
  - Severe bleeding (as evaluated by clinician).
- Severe organ involvement:
  - Aspartate aminotransferase (AST) or alanine aminotransferase (ALT) ≥1000 units/L/ Impaired consciousness/organ failure.

KEY POINTS

- Dengue is an arboviral disease that is similar to the chikungunya and Zika viruses.
- It is a common infection in the febrile returning traveller.
- Severe headache with rash and fever are common symptoms with dengue.
- Severe dengue is more likely in patients who have had previous dengue infection.
- Dengue fever can become severe and require ICU support due to plasma leakage.
- Management of dengue is supportive.

CASE 84: REDNESS AND SWELLING IN ARMS

History

A 24-year-old man presents to the hospital with rapid spreading redness of his left arm. It has progressed from his hand to his elbow within hours. He mentions a recent puncture wound on his left hand from gardening, but otherwise was fit and well prior to this illness.

Examination

He looks very unwell. His left arm is swollen and hot and is exquisitely tender to touch. There is some bruising around the puncture site. He is tachycardic, with a low blood pressure and normal oxygen saturations. His respiratory and cardiovascular examinations are normal.

INVESTIGATIONS

		Normal
Haemoglobin	13.8 g/dL	13.3–17.7 g/dL
White cell count	20.8×10^9/L	$3.9–10.6 \times 10^9$/L
Platelets	600×10^9/L	$150–440 \times 10^9$/L
Lactate	5	<2.0
Creatine kinase	600	
C-reactive protein (CRP)	250 mg/L	<5 mg/L
Blood film: Left shift		

QUESTIONS

- What are your differentials in this patient?
- What investigations are indicated?
- How would you manage this patient?

ANSWER 84

This gentleman has a rapidly progressing cellulitis which is exquisitely tender. Given the findings of rapid progression, severe pain and systemic features, this is very concerning for necrotising fasciitis.

Necrotising fasciitis is an infection that affects the deep soft tissues, resulting in destruction of the muscle fascia and subcutaneous fat, and spreads quickly in areas of poor blood supply. Depending on the body site affected, it may have different names (e.g., infection of the penis, scrotum and perineum is known as Fournier's gangrene). It can be divided into two microbiological types:

- **Type 1, polymicrobial:** Often caused by aerobic (e.g., *Escherichia coli, Enterobacter*) and anaerobic bacteria (*Clostridioides, Bacteroides, etc.*) together, depending on the site of infection.
- **Type 2, monomicrobial:** Often caused by Group A *Streptococcus* (GAS) or other *beta haemolytic Streptococcus* or *Staphylococcus aureus*.

Laboratory findings include elevated inflammatory markers, acute kidney injury, elevations in creatinine kinase (due to muscle death) and increased lactate. Patients should be managed as per sepsis guidance with prompt blood cultures, fluid resuscitation, frequent monitoring of the vital signs and intensive care unit review as needed.

Suspicion of necrotising fasciitis should prompt immediate surgical referral, as the most important aspect of management is urgent, aggressive debridement of necrotic tissue.

Antibiotic guidance should be sought from the local microbiology team. Generally, a broad-spectrum antibiotic which covers gram-positive, gram-negative and anaerobic bacteria, such as piperacillin-tazobactam, is advised. Clindamycin is often prescribed in addition, as it has been shown to counteract toxins produced by GAS. Linezolid is an alternative to clindamycin. An aminoglycoside such as gentamicin may be added for patients who are shocked.

Intravenous immunoglobulin is sometimes given in severe disease, based on toxin neutralising activity against streptococcal toxic shock syndrome.

In this patient, the source of the infection is possibly through his cut from gardening, which proceeded to cause cellulitis and then necrotising fasciitis. Group A *streptococcus (Streptococcus pyogenes)* is a gram-positive coccus, which is a very virulent organism. It commonly causes pharyngitis, but other syndromes include a range of skin and soft tissue infections from impetigo to erysipelas, cellulitis, abscesses and necrotising soft-tissue infections. Other infections include toxic shock syndrome and puerperal sepsis. Poststreptococcal complications such as rheumatic fever and glomerulonephritis may occur.

 KEY POINTS

- Group A *Streptococcus* can cause rapidly progressive infections.
- Commonly, it causes sore throat.
- Necrotising fasciitis can be polymicrobial or monomicrobial.
- Necrotising fasciitis needs urgent surgical review for debridement.

Section 10
GASTROENTEROLOGY

CASE 85: GENERAL WEAKNESS

History

An 82-year-old man is sent to the emergency department by his general practitioner (GP). The man is complaining of weakness and general malaise. He has complained of general pains in the muscles, and he also has some pains in the joints, particularly the elbows, wrists and knees. Three weeks earlier, he fell and hit his leg and has some local pain related to this.

He is a non-smoker who does not drink any alcohol and has not been on any medication. Twelve years ago, he had a myocardial infarction and was put on a beta-blocker, but he has not had a prescription for this in the past 6 years. Twenty years ago, he had a cholecystectomy. He used to work as a labourer until his retirement at the age of 63.

He lives alone in a second-floor flat. His wife died 5 years ago. He has one son who lives in Ireland and whom he has not seen for 3 years.

Examination

He is tender over the muscles around his limb girdles and there is a little tenderness over the elbows, wrists and knees. The mouth looks normal except that his tongue appears rather smooth. He has no teeth and has lost his dentures. There are no other abnormalities to find in the cardio-vascular, respiratory or alimentary systems. In the legs, he has a superficial laceration on the front of the right shin. This is oozing blood and has not healed. There is a petechial rash around the ankles. There are some larger areas of bruising on the arms and the legs, which he says have not been associated with any trauma.

🔍 INVESTIGATIONS

		Normal
Haemoglobin	10.1 g/dL	13.7–17.7 g/dL
Mean corpuscular volume (MCV)	74 fL	80–99 fL
White cell count	7.9×10^9/L	$3.9–10.6 \times 10^9$/L
Neutrophils	6.3×10^9/L	$1.8–7.7 \times 10^9$/L
Lymphocytes	1.2×10^9/L	$1.0–4.8 \times 10^9$/L
Platelets	334×10^9/L	$150–440 \times 10^9$/L

❓ QUESTIONS

- What essential area of the history is not covered?
- What are the key signs to consider in this presentation?
- What is the likely diagnosis?

ANSWER 85

A dietary history is an essential part of any history and is particularly important here; a number of features point towards a possible nutritional problem. He has been a widower for five years, with no family support. He lives alone on a second-floor flat, which may make it difficult for him to get out. He has lost his dentures, which likely makes it difficult for him to eat. The easiest way may be to ask him to tell you what he eats in a typical day and his food intake in the last 48 hours.

He has a petechial rash, which could be related to coagulation problems, but the platelet count is normal. It would be important to examine the rash carefully to see if it is distributed around the hair follicles. A number of features suggest a possible diagnosis of scurvy from vitamin C deficiency. Body stores of vitamin C are sufficient to last 2–3 months. The rash, muscle and joint pains and tenderness, poor wound healing and microcytic anaemia are all features of scurvy. The classic feature of bleeding from the gums would not be present in an edentulous patient.

Plasma measurements of vitamin C are difficult because of the wide range in normal subjects. In this patient, replacement with ascorbic acid orally cleared up the symptoms within 2 weeks. It would be important to look for other nutritional deficiencies in this situation and to arrange support to ensure that the situation did not recur after his discharge from the hospital.

 KEY POINTS

- A nutritional history should be part of any clinical assessment, particularly in the elderly.
- Vitamin deficiencies can occur in patients on a poor diet in the absence of any problem with malabsorption.

CASE 86: ABDOMINAL PAIN

History

A 44-year-old woman presents to her general practitioner (GP) complaining of pain in her epigastrium radiating into her back. The pain developed 18 hours earlier and has become progressively more severe. She has not eaten for the last 24 hours and has vomited altered food and then fluid, but no blood, on 4 occasions. She has had some looseness of her bowel motions.

She feels feverish and increasingly unwell. She has no pain on passing urine and no urinary frequency. Her last menstrual period was 2 weeks ago.

She had similar but much milder pains a few months ago. She has no other significant past medical history.

She smokes 15–20 cigarettes per day and drinks around half a bottle of wine each night. She has not used any recreational drugs.

Examination

She looks unwell. Her temperature is 38.8°C. Her pulse rate is 110/min, and blood pressure is 102/64 mmHg. In the respiratory system, there is some dullness to percussion at the left base. She is tender to palpation in the epigastrium and the centre of the abdomen. There is some guarding and rebound tenderness around the umbilicus. There is a suggestion of some skin discolouration in the flanks. Bowel sounds are sparse. Rectal examination is normal; there is some brown poorly formed stool on the examination glove.

🔍 INVESTIGATIONS

		Normal
Haemoglobin	15.3 g/dL	11.7–15.7 g/dL
White cell count	15.2 × 10⁹/L	3.5–11.0 × 10⁹/L
Platelets	412 × 10⁹/L	150–440 × 10⁹/L
Sodium	140 mmol/L	135–145 mmol/L
Potassium	3.5 mmol/L	3.5–5.0 mmol/L
Urea	9.3 mmol/L	2.5–6.7 mmol/L
Creatinine	82 μmol/L	70–120 μmol/L
C-reactive protein (CRP)	192 mg/L	<5 mg/L

Urinalysis: trace protein; trace blood; nitrites negative
Chest radiograph: small left-side pleural effusion
Abdominal radiograph: normal

❓ QUESTIONS

- What is the diagnosis?
- How would you assess and investigate this patient?
- How would you manage this patient?

ANSWER 86

The most likely diagnosis is acute pancreatitis. This most commonly presents with central or epigastric pain which radiates to the back. A posteriorly perforating duodenal ulcer may produce a similar pattern of pain. Nausea, vomiting and fever are common and fluid loss leads to haemodynamic instability and shock. The tachycardia, low blood pressure and haemoconcentration suggest fluid depletion. On examination, there are signs of peritonitis. In severe cases of acute pancreatitis, haemorrhage may produce blood staining in the skin of the flanks (Grey-Turner's sign) or around the umbilicus (Cullen's sign). Pleural effusions may occur, especially on the left, or pulmonary oedema. The raised white count and high CRP reflect the associated severe inflammation in acute pancreatitis.

The most common precipitating causes of acute pancreatitis are excessive alcohol use and gallstones, which account for 75% of cases. Other less common causes are hypercalcaemia, hyperlipidaemia, abdominal trauma, drugs such as corticosteroids, diuretics, pentamidine, azathioprine, infections such as mumps, coxsackie virus and cytomegalovirus.

Diagnosis is based on the clinical picture and raised levels of serum amylase or lipase. Elevations of amylase can occur also in mesenteric ischaemia and other acute abdominal conditions but an amylase more than three times the upper limit of normal with typical clinical features is diagnostic. Imaging such as computed tomography (CT) scan can show inflammation in the pancreas but is not usually necessary. Ultrasound may show underlying biliary tract disease but is less sensitive in the setting of acute pancreatitis. Magnetic resonance cholangiopancreatography (MRCP) can also be used in the diagnosis of suspected biliary and pancreatic duct obstruction.

Various staging criteria have been used to grade the severity of acute pancreatitis. The Ransom criteria are widely used for alcohol-induced disease, applied up to 48 hours after onset:

On admission:
- >55 years
- WBC count >16 × 10⁹/L
- Blood glucose >10 mmol/L
- Serum LDH >350 IU/L
- AST level >250 IU/L

Up to 48 hours:
- Haematocrit fall >10%
- Urea increased >1.8 mmol/L
- Serum calcium <2.0 mmol/L
- p_aO_2 <8.0 kPa
- Base deficit >4 mEq/L
- Estimated fluid sequestration >600 mL

With one point for each item, a score of >2 is predictive of severe pancreatitis and warrants admission to the intensive care unit. Alternative scores such as the Glasgow criteria are often used.

Management is predominantly fluid replacement and analgesia while keeping the patient nil by mouth. There is often considerable fluid loss retro- and intraperitoneally. Antibiotic treatment is still uncertain and is not routinely used.

Systemic complications may be related to inflammation and fluid loss, acute respiratory distress syndrome, multiple organ dysfunction or pancreatic damage producing diabetes. Hypocalcaemia may occur as calcium is involved in saponification of fats retroperitoneally. Local complications are related to pancreatic necrosis, secondary infection and development of pancreatic pseudocysts.

! DIFFERENTIAL DIAGNOSIS OF ACUTE PANCREATITIS

Other conditions to consider are:
- Pancreatic pseudocyst
- Pancreatic dysfunction (diabetes mellitus; malabsorption due to exocrine failure)
- Pancreatic cancer

Although these are common symptoms, they are not always present. Simple abdominal pain may be the sole symptom. The most common causes are:
- Alcohol
- Gallstones
- Metabolic disorders: Hereditary pancreatitis, hypercalcemia, hyperlipidaemia, malnutrition
- Abdominal trauma
- Penetrating ulcers
- Malignancy
- Drugs: Steroids, sulfonamides, furosemide, thiazides
- Infections: Mumps, coxsackie virus, mycoplasma pneumoniae, ascaris, clonorchis
- Structural abnormalities: Choledochocele, pancreas divisum

🔑 KEY POINTS

- The common causes of acute pancreatitis are alcohol and gallstone disease.
- The diagnosis of acute pancreatitis relies on the clinical picture and serum amylase or lipase.
- Adequate fluid replacement is an important part of management.

CASE 87: ABDOMINAL DISCOMFORT

History

A 64-year-old woman with a 6-month history of mild abdominal discomfort is referred to the Gastroenterology clinic. This discomfort has been intermittent and involved the right iliac fossa mainly. There has been no particular relation to eating or to bowel movements. Over this time, her appetite has gone down a little, and she thinks that she has lost around 5 kg in weight. The intensity of the pain has become slightly worse over this time, and it is now present on most days.

Over the past 6 weeks, she has developed some new symptoms. She has developed a different sort of cramping abdominal pain mainly in the right iliac fossa. This pain has been associated with a feeling of the need to defaecate and often with some diarrhoea. During these episodes, her husband has commented that she looked red in the face, but she has associated this with the abdominal discomfort and the embarrassment from the urgent need to have her bowels open.

There is no other relevant previous medical history. She has smoked 15 cigarettes daily for the last 45 years, and she drinks about 7 units of alcohol each week. She has noticed a little breathlessness on occasion over the past few months and has heard herself wheeze on several occasions. She has never had any problems with asthma, and there is no family history of asthma or other atopic conditions.

She worked as a school secretary for 30 years and has never had a job involving any industrial exposure. She has no pets. She has lived all her life in London, and her only trip outside the UK was a day trip to France.

> 🔍 **INVESTIGATIONS**
>
> A computed tomography (CT) scan of her abdomen was performed and is shown in Figure 87.1.

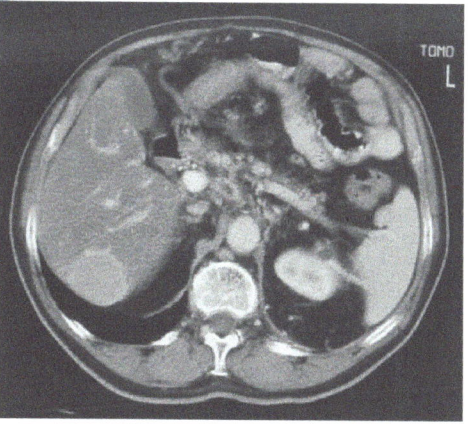

Figure 87.1 Computed tomography scan of the abdomen.

> ❓ **QUESTIONS**
>
> - What diagnoses should be considered?
> - What investigations should be performed?
> - How can symptoms be managed?

ANSWER 87

The symptoms she describes raise the possibility of a 5-hydroxytryptamine (5-HT)-secreting carcinoid tumour. The typical clinical features of the carcinoid syndrome are facial flushing, abdominal cramps and diarrhoea. Sometimes, there is asthma and right-sided heart valve problems. The symptoms are characteristically intermittent and may come at times of increased release on activity. Skin changes may be persistent.

The CT scan of the liver shows a space-occupying lesion in the liver likely to represent a metastasis to the liver. Fluid-containing cystic lesions are of lower density. Other secondary tumours would give a similar appearance. Carcinoids do not generally produce their symptoms until they have metastasised to the liver from their original site, which is usually in the small bowel. In the small bowel, tumours may produce local symptoms of obstruction or bleeding.

The symptoms of carcinoid tumours are related to the secretion of 5-HT by the tumour. The diagnosis depends on finding a high level of the metabolite 5-hydroxyindole acetic acid (5-HIAA) in a 24-h collection of urine. Histology can be obtained from a liver biopsy guided to the correct area by ultrasound or CT.

The symptoms can be controlled by antagonists of 5-HT, such as cyproheptadine, or by inhibitors of its synthesis (p-chlorophenylalanine) or release (octreotide). The tumour can be reduced in size with consequent lessening of symptoms by embolisation of its arterial supply using interventional radiology techniques.

When odd symptoms such as those described here occur, the diagnosis of carcinoid tumour should always be remembered and investigated. Most of the investigations for suspected carcinoid turn out to be negative.

Carcinoid tumours can occur in the lung where they act as slowly growing malignant tumours. From the lung, they can eventually be associated with left heart-valve problems. The other typical carcinoid features occur only after metastasis to the liver.

 KEY POINTS

- Intermittent skin flushing, diarrhoea, wheezing and abdominal cramps are symptoms of the carcinoid syndrome.
- All these symptoms have much commoner causes.
- Metastasis to the liver is present before the symptoms of carcinoid syndrome occur.

CASE 88: CHEST PAIN

History

A 64-year-old woman has a 10-year history of retrosternal pain. The pain is often present in bed at night and may be precipitated by bending down. Occasionally, the pain comes on after eating and, on some occasions, it appears to have been precipitated by exercise. The pain has been described as having a burning and a tight quality to it. The pain is not otherwise exacerbated by respiratory movements or position.

Her husband has angina, and on one occasion she took one of his glyceryl trinitrate tablets. She thinks that this probably helped her pain since it seemed to stop a little faster than usual. She has also bought some indigestion tablets from a local pharmacy and thinks that these probably helped also.

Examination

She is 1.62 m (5 ft., 4 in.) tall and weighs 82 kg, giving her a body mass index of 31.3 kg/m² (recommended range 20–25 kg/m²). No abnormalities are found in the cardiovascular, respiratory or gastrointestinal systems.

🔍 **INVESTIGATIONS**

Her chest radiograph is normal, and the electrocardiogram (ECG) is shown in Figure 88.1. She had an exercise ECG performed, and she was able to perform 8 minutes of exercise. Her heart rate went up to 130/min with no change in the ST segments on the ECG and normal heart and blood pressure responses.
The haemoglobin, renal and liver functions are normal.

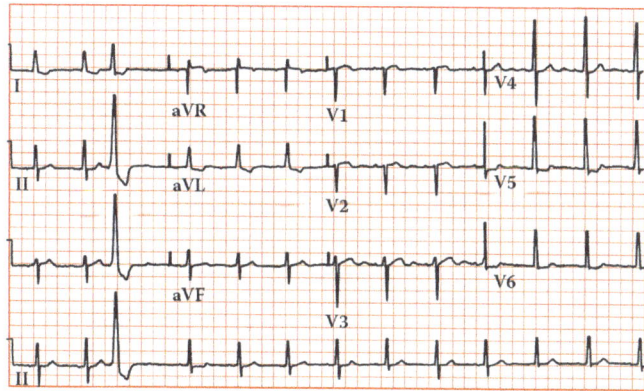

Figure 88.1 Electrocardiogram.

❓ **QUESTIONS**

- What is the likely diagnosis?
- What would be appropriate management?
- What further investigations may be useful?

ANSWER 88

A number of features in the history make oesophageal reflux a likely diagnosis. The character and position of the pain and the relation to lying flat and to bending mean reflux is more likely. She is overweight, increasing the likelihood of reflux. The improvement with glyceryl trinitrate and with proprietary antacids is inconclusive. The ECG shows one ventricular ectopic and some T-wave changes in leads I, aVl, V5 and V6, which would be compatible with myocardial ischaemia but are not specific. The exercise ECG was negative, which reduces the likelihood of ischaemic heart disease, although it certainly does not rule it out. Other causes of chest pain are less likely with the length of history.

In view of the long history and the features suggesting oesophageal reflux, it would be reasonable to initiate a trial of therapy for oesophageal reflux with regular antacid therapy, H_2-receptor blockers or a proton pump inhibitor (omeprazole or lansoprazole). If the pain responds to this form of therapy, then additional actions such as weight loss (she is well above ideal body weight) and raising the head of the bed at night should be added. If doubt remains, a barium swallow should show the tendency to reflux, and a gastroscopy would show evidence of oesophagitis. There is a broad association between the presence of oesophageal reflux, evidence of oesophagitis at endoscopy and biopsy and the symptoms of heartburn. However, each can occur independently of the others.

Recording of pH in the oesophagus over 24 h can provide additional useful information. It is achieved by passing a small pH-sensitive electrode into the oesophagus through the nose. This provides an objective measure of the amount of acid reaching the oesophagus and the times when this occurs.

This woman had an endoscopy that showed oesophagitis, and treatment with omeprazole and an alginate relieved her symptoms. Attempts at weight loss were not successful.

 KEY POINTS

- The oesophagus is a common source of non-specific chest pain with a normal ECG.
- A 24-h pH recording in the oesophagus provides further information on acid reflux.

CASE 89: ACUTE DIARRHOEA

History

A 74-year-old woman is admitted to hospital from a residential care home with abdominal pains. She is passing stool normally. She has a history of dementia and gastro-oesophageal reflux. She takes lansoprazole daily. On examination, she is tender in the left iliac fossa. A computed tomography (CT) scan of her abdomen confirms the suspicion of diverticulitis and she is treated with intravenous cefuroxime.

Her symptoms resolve and she makes a good recovery, but just prior to discharge, she has an episode of diarrhoea. The next day, she has 4 episodes of watery diarrhoea and complains of new crampy abdominal pain.

Examination

On examination, her mucous membranes are dry and she has a fever of 38.5°C. She has diffuse abdominal tenderness. There is no guarding or rebound tenderness. She has prominent bowel sounds.

INVESTIGATIONS		
		Normal
Haemoglobin	14.2 g/dL	11.7–15.7 g/dL
Mean corpuscular volume (MCV)	87 fL	80–99 fL
White cell count	16.3×10^9/L	$3.5–11.0 \times 10^9$/L
Platelets	324×10^9/L	$150–440 \times 10^9$/L
Sodium	134 mmol/L	135–145 mmol/L
Potassium	3.8 mmol/L	3.5–5.0 mmol/L
Urea	9.2 mmol/L	2.5–6.7 mmol/L
Creatinine	189 mmol/L	70–120 µmol/L

?	QUESTIONS

- What is the likely diagnosis?
- How would you further examine and investigate this patient?
- How would you manage this patient?

ANSWER 89

This patient has developed diarrhoea and abdominal discomfort following a course of intravenous broad-spectrum antibiotics. This raises the likelihood of infection with *Clostridium difficile*.

Risk factors include:

- **Her age:** 80% of *C. difficile* infections occur in people aged over 65 years. A lower density of gut bacteria in this age group facilitates colonisation by *C. difficile*.
- **The use of proton pump inhibitors:** Due to gastric acid suppression.
- **Long-term care facilities:** *C. difficile* spreads by faecal–oral routes and some studies suggest 10% of people residing in long-term care facilities are colonised with *C. difficile*.

Stool samples should be obtained from any hospital patient who has unexplained diarrhoea or diarrhoea and other risk factors.

Cases are defined and managed according to severity:

- **Mild:** Mild diarrhoea (fewer than 3 stools a day), normal white cell count.
- **Moderate:** Moderate diarrhoea (3–5 stools a day), white count may be raised but remains less than $15 \times 10^9/L$.
- **Severe:** A white cell count greater than $15 \times 10^9/L$, an acutely increased serum creatinine (>50% above baseline), a temperature over 38.5°C or clinical or radiological signs of severe colitis. Number of stools may be a less reliable indicator here.
- **Life threatening:** Hypotension, ileus or toxic megacolon or CT evidence of severe disease.

Mild, moderate and severe cases are treated with oral vancomycin. Oral vancomycin is not absorbed by the gut and will act locally on inflamed gut tissue to eradicate *C. difficile*, making it a safe and effective treatment. For life threatening infection, two agents are often used, oral vancomycin and intravenous metronidazole. All cases of *C. difficile* infection in hospitalised patients should be discussed with the microbiology or infectious diseases team.

This woman has evidence of at least severe disease and should be prescribed oral vancomycin. Additionally, CT imaging of the bowel should be requested. Essential areas of management are regular fluid status reviews, accurate recording of fluid balance and stool output, intravenous hydration, monitoring electrolytes and nutrition and monitoring for complications.

Another extremely important aspect is infection control. As soon as *C. difficile* infection is suspected, the patient should be isolated in a separate room and the infection control team is alerted to assess the situation and enforce infection control policies. *C. difficile* is an anaerobic spore forming gram-positive rod. Spores can persist in the hospital environment for long durations, making comprehensive infection control protocols a key part in managing outbreaks. Alcohol-based hand gels are not effective against *C. difficile* spores; therefore, soap and water must be used for handwashing during an outbreak. Injudicious use of antibiotics also leads to outbreaks; therefore, involvement of the microbiologist and reinforcement of antimicrobial stewardship is essential.

 KEY POINTS

- *C. difficile* infection should be suspected in any hospital patient who develops diarrhoea.
- A strict antibiotic policy, a high degree of suspicion and good infection control measures all help to reduce problems with *C. difficile* infection.

CASE 90: TIREDNESS

History

A 22-year-old woman complains of tiredness for 6 months. Her only other symptom is a gradual increase in frequency of bowel movements from once a day in her teens to 2–3 times daily. She has no abdominal pain and has no change in appetite. She says that the bowel movements can be difficult to flush away on occasions, but this is not a consistent problem. She is a non-smoker and drinks rarely. She has been a vegetarian for 5 years but eats dairy foods and fish regularly. She thinks that her grandmother, who lived in Ireland, had some bowel problems, but she died 3 years ago, at age 68. She is an infant-school teacher and spends a lot of her spare time in keep-fit classes and routines at a local gym. She enjoys her work and socialises regularly with a wide circle of friends.

Examination

She is 1.62 m (5 ft., 4 in.) tall and weighs 49 kg. She looks a little pale and thin. Examination of her abdomen showed no abnormalities, and there are no other significant abnormalities to find in any other system.

🔍 INVESTIGATIONS

		Normal
Haemoglobin	9.8 g/dL	11.7–15.7 g/dL
Mean corpuscular volume (MCV)	98 fL	80–99 fL
White cell count	6.5×10^9/L	$3.5–11.0 \times 10^9$/L
Platelets	247×10^9/L	$150–440 \times 10^9$/L
Red cell folate	44 mg/L	>160 mg/L
Vitamin B_{12}	280 ng/L	176–925 ng/L
Thyroid-stimulating hormone	3.5 mU/L	0.3–6.0 mU/L
Free thyroxine	12.9 pmol/L	9.0–22.0 pmol/L

The blood film is reported as a dimorphic film with remnants of nuclear material (Howell–Jolly bodies) in some of the red blood cells.

? QUESTIONS

- How do you interpret these findings?
- What is the likely diagnosis?
- How might this be confirmed?

DOI: 10.1201/9781003350934-100

ANSWER 90

The most likely diagnosis is malabsorption from coeliac disease. The report of a dimorphic blood film means that there are both small and large cells. This suggests that the anaemia is caused by a combination of the folate deficiency indicated by the red cell folate and by iron deficiency. The Howell–Jolly bodies are dark blue regular inclusions in the red cells that are typically found in the blood of patients after splenectomy or are associated with the splenic atrophy characteristic of coeliac disease. In coeliac disease, there is a sensitivity to dietary gluten, a water-insoluble protein found in many cereals. The proximal small bowel is the main site involved with loss of villi and an inflammatory infiltrate causing reduced absorption.

! CAUSES OF MACROCYTOSIS IN THE BLOOD FILM

- Folate deficiency
- Vitamin B$_{12}$ deficiency
- Excessive alcohol consumption
- Hypothyroidism
- Certain drugs (e.g., azathioprine, methotrexate)
- Primary acquired sideroblastic anaemia and myelodysplastic syndromes

---

Coeliac disease is made more likely by a possible positive family history and the origin from Ireland, where coeliac disease is four times as common as in the rest of the United Kingdom. Another diagnosis that might be considered is anorexia nervosa (her age and sex, commitment to exercise); she does not appear depressed (a common cause of weight loss and bowel disturbance) and the laboratory findings clearly indicate physical disease.

Diagnosis of coeliac disease can be confirmed by endoscopy, at which a biopsy can be taken from the distal duodenum. Typically, this will show complete villus atrophy. Immunoglobulin A (IgA) anti-tissue transglutaminase and IgA endomysial antibodies are usually positive when the patient is still in a gluten-containing diet and are a useful screening test. Treatment is a gluten-free diet with a repeat of the biopsy some months later to show improvement in the height of the villi in the small bowel. In some cases, temporary treatment with steroids may be needed to help recovery. A common cause of failure to recover the villus architecture is poor compliance to the difficult dietary constraints. Symptoms may persist if patients have lactose intolerance or irritable bowel syndrome.

🔑 KEY POINTS

- Howell–Jolly bodies are characteristic of hyposplenism.
- Coeliac disease can present at any age with non-specific symptoms; absence of abdominal pain or steatorrhoea are not unusual.
- Typical features of fat malabsorption may not be evident if the patient eats a diet with little or no fat intake.

CASE 91: RECURRENT CHEST INFECTIONS

History

A 45-year-old woman is admitted to hospital with pneumonia. She has had 3 episodes of cough, fever and purulent sputum over the last 6 months. One of these was associated with right-sided pleuritic chest pain. These have been treated at home by her general practitioner (GP). In addition, she has a 5-year history of difficulty with swallowing. Initially this was mild, but it has become progressively worse. She says that food seems to stick in the low retrosternal area. This applies to all types of solid food. She has lost 5 kg in weight over the past 2 months. Sometimes, the difficulty with swallowing seems to improve during a meal. Recently, she has had trouble with regurgitation and vomiting of recognisable food.

Three years ago, her GP arranged for an outpatient upper gastrointestinal endoscopy, which was normal. She was reassured, but the problem has increased in severity. There is no other relevant medical history or family history. She lived in the northwestern coast of the United States for 4 years until 10 years ago. She works as a shop assistant. She has never smoked and drinks less than 5 units of alcohol each week. There has been no disturbance of micturition. She has always tended to be constipated, and this has been a little worse recently.

Examination

She looks thin. In the respiratory system, there are some crackles at the right base. There are no abnormalities in the cardiovascular system, abdomen or other systems.

 INVESTIGATIONS

Her chest radiograph is shown in Figure 91.1.

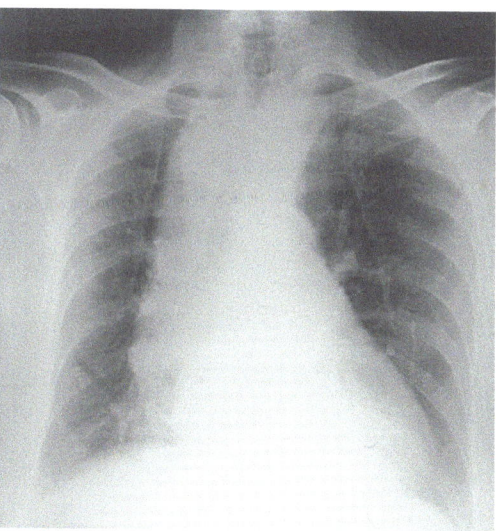

Figure 91.1 Chest Radiograph. (From Curtis and Whitehouse, *Radiology for the MRCP*, Arnold, London, 1998.)

? **QUESTIONS**

- What is the likely diagnosis?
- How would you establish this?
- What are some common causes of this condition?

ANSWER 91

The likely diagnosis is achalasia of the cardia, a primary neurological disturbance of the nerve plexuses at the lower end of the oesophagus. The radiograph shows a dilated, fluid-filled oesophagus with no visible gastric air bubble. Endoscopy may be normal in the early stages, as in this case. The oesophagus has now dilated, and there has been spillover of stagnant food into the lungs, giving her the episodes of repeated respiratory infections. Such aspiration is most likely to affect the right lower lobe because of the more vertical right main bronchus, although the result of aspiration at night may depend on the position of the patient. The dysphagia is often variable early on. It tends to be present for all foods, indicating a motility problem, and there may initially be some relief from the mechanical load as the oesophagus fills. Dysphagia for bulky, solid foods first usually indicates an obstructive lesion.

The diagnosis can be made at this stage by a barium swallow showing the dilated oesophagus. Earlier, it may have required careful cine-radiology with a bolus of food impregnated with barium or oesophageal motility studies using a catheter fitted with pressure sensors to detect the abnormal motility of the oesophageal muscle.

A similar condition can be produced by the protozoan parasite *Trypanosoma cruzi* (Chagas disease), but this is limited to South and Central America, and would not be relevant to her stay in the northwest United States.

Other common causes of dysphagia are benign oesophageal structures from acid reflux, malignant structures, external compression or an oesophageal pouch. Achalasia may be managed by muscle relaxants when mild, but often requires treatment to disrupt the lower oesophageal muscle by endoscopic dilation or surgery.

 KEY POINTS

- The subjective site of blockage in dysphagia may not reflect accurately the level of the obstruction.
- Persistent dysphagia without explanation needs investigation by barium swallow or endoscopy.

CASE 92: WEIGHT LOSS

History

A 67-year-old man attends his general practitioner's (GP's) surgery. He says that he has lost 10 kg in weight over the past 4 months. This has been associated with a decrease in appetite and an increasing problem with vomiting. The vomiting has been productive of food eaten many hours previously. During the last month, he has noticed some weakness, particularly in his legs, climbing hills and stairs.

He is a smoker of 20 cigarettes per day and drinks about 10 units of alcohol each week. There is no relevant family history. His past medical history consists of hypertension, which was treated for 2 years with beta-blockers. He stopped taking these 4 months ago.

Examination

He looks thin and unwell. His pulse is 82/min. His blood pressure is 148/86 mmHg. No abnormalities are found on examination of the cardiovascular and respiratory systems. There are no masses to feel in the abdomen and no tenderness, but a succussion splash is present.

INVESTIGATIONS		
		Normal
Sodium	130 mmol/L	135–145 mmol/L
Potassium	3.0 mmol/L	3.5–5.0 mmol/L
Chloride	82 mmol/L	95–105 mmol/L
Bicarbonate	41 mmol/L	25–35 mmol/L
Urea	15.6 mmol/L	2.5–6.7 mmol/L
Creatinine	100 µmol/L	76–120 µmol/L
Calcium	2.38 mmol/L	2.12–2.65 mmol/L
Phosphate	1.16 mmol/L	0.8–1.45 mmol/L
Alkaline phosphatase	128 IU/L	30–300 IU/L
Alanine aminotransferase	32 IU/L	5–35 IU/L
Gamma-glutamyl transpeptidase	38 IU/L	11–51 IU/L

Full blood count: normal

Chest radiograph: clear

? QUESTIONS

- What is the likely explanation for these findings?
- What is the most likely diagnosis?
- What are the next steps in management?

DOI: 10.1201/9781003350934-102

267

ANSWER 92

The clinical picture suggests obstruction to outflow from the stomach. This would be compatible with vomiting of residual food some time after eating and the succussion splash from the retained fluid and food in the stomach. The biochemical results fit with this diagnosis. There is a rise in urea but not creatinine, suggesting a degree of dehydration. Sodium, chloride and hydrogen ions are lost in the vomited stomach contents. Loss of hydrochloric acid produces metabolic alkalosis. In compensation, hydrogen ions are retained by the exchange for potassium in the kidney and across the cell membranes, leading to hypokalaemia, and carbonic acid dissociates to hydrogen ions and bicarbonate. The hypokalaemia indicates considerable loss of total body potassium, which is mostly in the skeletal muscle, and explains the patient's recent weakness.

The most likely cause would be a carcinoma of the stomach involving the pyloric antrum and producing obstruction to outflow. A chronic gastric ulcer in this area could produce the same picture from associated scarring, and gastroscopy and biopsy would be necessary to be sure of the diagnosis.

Gastroscopy may be difficult because of retained food in the stomach. In this case, after the stomach was washed out, a tumour was visible at the pylorus, causing almost complete obstruction of the outflow tract of the stomach. The next step would be a computed tomography (CT) scan of the abdomen to look for metastases in the liver and any suggestion of local spread of the tumour outside the stomach. If there is no evidence of extension or spread, or even to relieve obstruction, laparotomy and resection should be considered. Otherwise, chemotherapy and surgical palliation are treatment options.

 KEY POINTS

- Vomiting food eaten a long time previously suggests gastric outlet obstruction.
- Mild-to-moderate dehydration tends to increase urea more than creatinine.
- Prolonged vomiting causes a typical picture of hypochloraemic metabolic alkalosis.
- Carcinoma of the stomach can present without abdominal pain or anaemia.

CASE 93: DIARRHOEA

History

A 35-year-old woman has a year-long history of intermittent diarrhoea, which has never been bad enough for her to seek medical help in the past. However, she has become much worse over 1 week, with episodes of bloody diarrhoea 10 times a day. She has had some crampy lower abdominal pain, which lasts for 1–2 h and is partially relieved by defaecation. Over the past 2–3 days, she has become weak with the persistent diarrhoea, and her abdomen has become more painful and bloated over the past 24 h.

She has no relevant previous medical history. Up to 1 year ago, her bowels were regular. There is no disturbance of micturition or menstruation. In her family history, she thinks one of her maternal aunts may have had bowel problems. She has two children, aged 3 and 8 years, who are both well. She travelled to Spain on holiday 6 months ago, but has not travelled elsewhere.

She smokes 10 cigarettes a day and drinks rarely. She took 2 days of amoxicillin after the diarrhoea began with no improvement or worsening of her bowels.

Examination

Her blood pressure is 108/66 mmHg. Her pulse rate is 110/min; respiratory rate is 18/min. Her abdomen is rather distended and tender generally, particularly in the left iliac fossa. Faint bowel sounds are audible.

🔍 INVESTIGATIONS

		Normal
Haemoglobin	11.1 g/dL	11.7–15.7 g/dL
Mean corpuscular volume (MCV)	79 fL	80–99 fL
White cell count	8.8×10^9/L	$3.5–11.0 \times 10^9$/L
Platelets	280×10^9/L	$150–440 \times 10^9$/L
Sodium	139 mmol/L	135–145 mmol/L
Potassium	3.3 mmol/L	3.5–5.0 mmol/L
Urea	7.6 mmol/L	2.5–6.7 mmol/L
Creatinine	89 µmol/L	70–120 µmol/L

The abdominal radiograph shows a dilated colon with no faeces.

❓ QUESTIONS

- What is your interpretation of these results?
- What is the likely diagnosis?
- What should be the management?

ANSWER 93

Bloody diarrhoea 10 times a day suggests serious active colitis. In the absence of any recent foreign travel, it is most likely that this is an acute episode of ulcerative colitis on top of chronic involvement. The dilated colon suggests a diagnosis of toxic megacolon, which can rupture with potentially fatal consequences. Investigations such as sigmoidoscopy and colonoscopy may be dangerous in this acute situation and should be deferred until there has been reasonable improvement. The blood results show mild microcytic anaemia, suggesting chronic blood loss, low potassium from diarrhoea (explaining in part her weakness) and raised urea, but normal creatinine, from loss of water and electrolytes.

If the history was just the acute symptoms, then infective causes of diarrhoea would be higher in the differential diagnosis. Nevertheless, stool should be examined for ova, parasites and culture. Inflammatory bowel disorders have a familial incidence, but the patient's aunt has an unknown condition, and the relationship is not close enough to be helpful in diagnosis. Smoking is associated with Crohn's disease, but ulcerative colitis is more common in non-smokers.

Although amoxicillin treatment can be associated with bowel disturbance or even *Clostridium difficile* infection, it is not relevant here since the diarrhoea was present before taking amoxicillin and did not change afterwards.

She should be treated immediately with corticosteroids and intravenous fluid replacement, including potassium. If the colon is increasing in size or is initially larger than 5.5 cm in diameter, then surgical consultation for possible laparotomy to prevent perforation should be pursued. If not, the steroids should be continued until the symptoms resolve and diagnostic procedures such as colonoscopy and biopsy can be carried out safely. Sulphasalazine or mesalazine are used in the chronic maintenance treatment of ulcerative colitis after resolution of the acute attack.

In this case, the colon steadily enlarged despite fluid replacement and other appropriate treatment. She required surgery with a total colectomy and ileorectal anastomosis. The histology confirmed ulcerative colitis. The ileorectal anastomosis will be reviewed regularly; there is an increased risk of rectal carcinoma.

 KEY POINTS

- Bloody diarrhoea implies serious colonic pathology.
- It is important to monitor colonic dilatation carefully in colitis, and vital to operate before rupture.
- Both Crohn's disease and ulcerative colitis can cause a similar picture of active colitis.

CASE 94: ABDOMINAL PAIN

History

A 38-year-old man has a 2-month history of abdominal pain. The pain is epigastric or central and is intermittent. He had a similar episode a year before. On that occasion, he took some indigestion mixture obtained from a retail pharmacy and the symptoms resolved after 10 weeks. The pain usually lasts for 30–60 min. It often occurs at night, when it can wake him up, and seems to improve after meals. Some foods, such as curries and other spicy foods, seem to cause the pain on occasions.

He has smoked 10–15 cigarettes per day for 25 years and drinks around 30 units of alcohol each week. He is not taking any medication at present. There is no other relevant medical history. He works as a financial broker in the city. He has been feeling more tired recently and had attributed this to the pressure of work. A blood count was sent.

Examination

There is mild tenderness in the epigastrium, but no other abnormalities.

INVESTIGATIONS

		Normal
Haemoglobin	10.2 g/dL	13.3–17.7 g/dL
Red cell count	6.4×10^{12}/L	$4.4–5.9 \times 10^{12}$/L
Mean corpuscular volume (MCV)	71 fL	80–99 fL
White cell count	8.9×10^9/L	$3.9–10.6 \times 10^9$/L
Platelets	350×10^9/L	$150–440 \times 10^9$/L
Iron	4 mmol/L	14–31 mmol/L
Total iron-binding capacity	76 mmol/L	45–70 mmol/L
Ferritin	6 mg/L	20–300 mg/L

The blood film is reported as showing microcytic, hypochromic red cells.

QUESTIONS

- How do you interpret these findings?
- What is the likely diagnosis?
- How should it be confirmed?

DOI: 10.1201/9781003350934-104

ANSWER 94

The blood count shows anaemia with a low MCV, indicating a microcytic anaemia. The high red cell count with low haemoglobin shows that the haemoglobin content of the cells is reduced. The low serum iron and ferritin with a high total iron-binding capacity (TIBC) confirm that this is related to true iron deficiency. The blood film confirms that the cells are microcytic and low in haemoglobin (hypochromasia). In anaemia of chronic disease, the cells may be microcytic and serum iron low, but the TIBC would be low also and ferritin normal. The diagnosis is most likely to be a peptic ulcer.

The commonest cause of iron-deficiency anaemia in a man is gastrointestinal blood loss. In a premenopausal woman, menstrual blood loss is the commonest cause. The abdominal pains would be consistent with those from a peptic ulcer, especially a duodenal ulcer when there is more often some relief from food. The diagnosis should be established by endoscopy because alternative diagnoses such as carcinoma of the stomach cannot be ruled out from the history. The site of the blood loss causing the iron deficiency should be established. At the same time, the presence of *Helicobacter pylori* should be investigated.

In this case, an endoscopy confirmed an active duodenal ulcer, and samples were positive for *H. pylori*. This is associated with gastritis and more than 90% of duodenal ulcers. Tests of expired breath and serum antibodies are alternative diagnostic tests. The *H. pylori* was treated by a combined regimen of omeprazole for 6 weeks and triple therapy with lansoprazole, amoxicillin and clarithromycin for 7 days. For small (<1 cm) uncomplicated ulcers, there is no indication for continuing proton pump inhibitors after completion of the course of antibiotics. By contrast, continuing antisecretory therapy until the cure of *H. pylori* is confirmed is important for complicated ulcers. He was given strong recommendations to stop smoking and to address his excessive alcohol consumption. The importance of stress as a risk factor for peptic ulcer disease remains controversial. The iron deficiency was corrected by additional oral iron, which was continued for 3 months to replenish the iron stores in the bone marrow. Patients with uncomplicated duodenal ulcers who have been treated do not need further endoscopy unless symptoms persist.

KEY POINTS

- Various antibiotic regimes have been shown to temporarily remove *H. pylori* and prevent or postpone recurrence of symptoms and ulceration.
- Replenishment of iron stores in the bone marrow needs 3 months of treatment with oral iron after the haemoglobin has returned to normal.
- Ferritin is an acute-phase protein and will be raised in the presence of acute illness even in the presence of iron deficiency.

CASE 95: ABDOMINAL PAIN

History

A 70-year-old woman is admitted to hospital with acute onset of abdominal pain. The abdominal pain started quite suddenly 24 h before admission and has continued since then. It is a constant central abdominal pain. She has vomited altered food on one occasion.

She has a history of occasional angina on exertion for 5 years. She has a glyceryl trinitrate spray, but she has not needed this in the past 3 months. A year ago, she was found to be in atrial fibrillation at 120/min and she was started on digoxin, which she still takes. The only other medical history of note is that she had a hysterectomy for menorrhagia 30 years ago and she has hypertension controlled on a small dose of a thiazide diuretic for the last 3 years. She does not take any other medication apart from low-dose aspirin. She does not smoke and does not drink alcohol. She retired from work as a cleaner 8 years ago.

Examination

She is in atrial fibrillation at a rate of 92/min with a blood pressure of 114/76 mmHg. Respiratory examination is normal. She is tender with some guarding in the centre of the abdomen. No masses are palpable in the abdomen, and there are just occasional bowel sounds to hear on auscultation. Over the next 2 h, her blood pressure falls to 84/60 mmHg and she is admitted to the intensive care unit (ICU) and monitored while initial investigations are performed. The abdominal radiograph shows no gas under the diaphragm and no dilated loops of bowel or fluid levels. While under observation, the urine output decreases. Re-examination showed that bowel sounds are now absent, though her hands and feet remain warm. Measurements of cardiac output in the ICU shows that it remains high.

🔍 **INVESTIGATIONS**

The observation charts are shown in Figure 95.1.

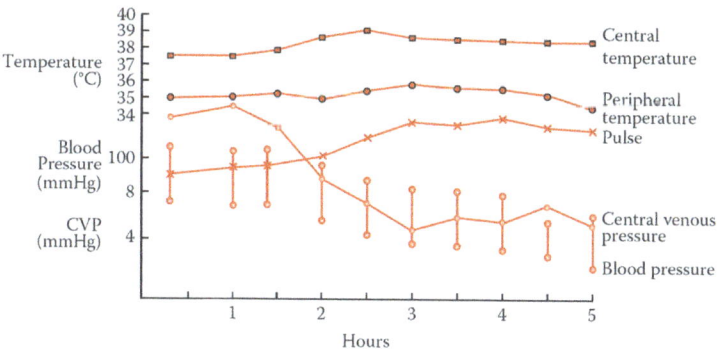

Figure 95.1 Chart from intensive care unit.

❓ **QUESTIONS**

- What is the likely cause of the abdominal pain?
- What further developments do the charts suggest?
- How should this patient be managed?

DOI: 10.1201/9781003350934-105

ANSWER 95

One diagnosis of the abdominal pain that would explain her condition and fit with her predisposing situation is ischaemic bowel caused by an embolus from the heart. The patient is likely to become very ill without markedly abnormal physical signs. Atrial fibrillation increases the likelihood of such an event. She has been on aspirin, which will reduce slightly the risk of embolic events, but is not on therapeutic anticoagulation, which would have decreased the risk further. In the presence of pre-existing cardiovascular problems, shown by the hypertension and angina, anticoagulation would normally be started if there are no contraindications. The risk of cerebrovascular accidents caused by emboli from the heart has been shown to be reduced. In lone atrial fibrillation with no underlying cardiac disease, the risks of emboli and the benefits of anticoagulation are less. There are alternative diagnoses, such as perforation or pancreatitis, and it is not possible to be sure of the cause of the abdominal problem from the information given here.

The chart of the observations (Figure 95.1) covers 5 hours. After the first hour or two, the central venous pressure drops, the blood pressure falls, and the pulse rate rises in association with the fall in urine output.

These findings show that she is developing shock with inadequate perfusion of vital organs.

> **! POSSIBLE CAUSES FOR SHOCK**
>
> | Types of shock | Example |
> | --- | --- |
> | Hypovolaemic shock | Blood loss |
> | Cardiogenic shock | Myocardial infarction |
> | Extracardiac obstructive shock | Pulmonary embolism |
> | Vasodilatory (distributive) shock | Sepsis |

All these causes are possible in this woman with abdominal problems and a history of ischaemic heart disease. The fact that the cardiac output is high makes blood loss and cardiogenic shock unlikely. The most likely cause is septic shock, for which peripheral vasodilation would lead to a high cardiac output but a falling blood pressure and rising pulse rate. Vasoconstriction and reduced blood flow occur in certain organs, such as the kidneys, leading to the term *distributive shock* with maintained overall cardiac output but inappropriate distribution of blood flow. The rise in central temperature and the lack of a marked fall in peripheral temperature would fit with this cause of the shock.

The patient was stabilised with fluid replacement and antibiotics before being taken for urgent surgery, where the diagnosis of ischaemic bowel from an embolus was confirmed. Arteriography can confirm the diagnosis, but confirmation is often at laparotomy, which is usually required to remove the necrotic bowel.

> **🔑 KEY POINTS**
>
> - Aspirin and anticoagulation should be considered in patients with atrial fibrillation.
> - Septic shock may be present with warm peripheries through vasodilation.
> - A drop in the central venous pressure may be the first sign of developing shock.

History

A 56-year-old woman presents to the emergency department complaining of abdominal pain. Twenty-four hours previously, she developed a continuous pain in the upper abdomen that has now worsened. The pain radiates into the back. She feels nauseated and alternately hot and cold. Her past medical history is notable for a duodenal ulcer, which was successfully treated with *Helicobacter* eradication therapy 5 years ago. She smokes 15 cigarettes a day and shares a bottle of wine each evening with her husband.

Examination

The patient looks unwell and dehydrated. She weighs 115 kg. She is febrile, 38.5°C, her pulse is 108/min and blood pressure is 124/76 mmHg. Cardiovascular and respiratory system examination is normal. She is tender in the right upper quadrant and epigastrium, with guarding and rebound tenderness. Bowel sounds are sparse.

🔍 INVESTIGATIONS

		Normal
Haemoglobin	14.7 g/dL	11.7–15.7 g/dL
White cell count	19.8×10^9/L	$3.5–11.0 \times 10^9$/L
Platelets	239×10^9/L	$150–440 \times 10^9$/L
Sodium	137 mmol/L	135–145 mmol/L
Potassium	4.8 mmol/L	3.5–5.0 mmol/L
Urea	8.6 mmol/L	2.5–6.7 mmol/L
Creatinine	116 µmol/L	70–120 µmol/L
Bilirubin	19 µmol/L	3–17 µmol/L
Alkaline phosphatase	58 IU/L	30–300 IU/L
Alanine aminotransferase (AAT)	67 IU/L	5–35 IU/L
Gamma-glutamyl transpeptidase	72 IU/L	11–51 IU/L
C-reactive protein (CRP)	256 mg/L	<5 mg/L

A plain abdominal radiograph is shown in Figure 96.1.

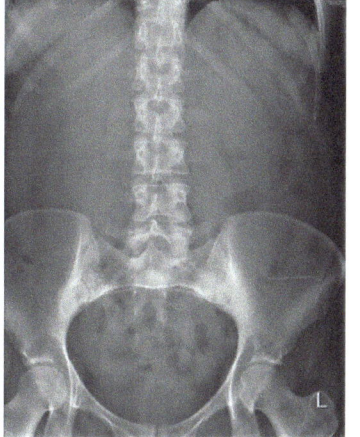

Figure 96.1 Plain abdominal radiograph.

❓ QUESTIONS

- What is the most likely diagnosis?
- What are the key signs to look out for in this condition?
- How would you manage this patient?

DOI: 10.1201/9781003350934-106

ANSWER 96

This woman has acute cholecystitis. Cholecystitis is most common in obese, middle-aged women. The pain is classically triggered by eating a fatty meal. Cholecystitis is usually caused by a gallstone impacting in the cystic duct. Continued secretion by the gallbladder leads to increased pressure and inflammation of the gallbladder wall. This can be complicated by bacterial infection most commonly due to Gram-negative organisms such as *Escherichia coli* and anaerobes. Ischaemia in the distended gallbladder can lead to perforation, causing either generalised peritonitis or formation of a localised abscess. Alternatively, the stone can spontaneously disimpact and the symptoms spontaneously improve. Gallstones can become stuck in the common bile duct, leading to cholangitis or pancreatitis. Rarely, gallstones can perforate through the inflamed gallbladder wall into the small intestine and cause intestinal obstruction (gallstone ileus).

The typical symptom of acute cholecystitis is sudden-onset right upper quadrant abdominal pain that radiates into the back. An episode of prolonged right-upper-quadrant pain associated with fever suggests acute cholecystitis rather than simple biliary colic. Jaundice usually occurs if there is a stone in the common bile duct.

There is usually fever, tachycardia, guarding and rebound tenderness in the right upper quadrant (Murphy's sign). In this patient, the leucocytosis and raised CRP are consistent with acute cholecystitis. If the serum bilirubin and liver enzymes are very deranged, acute cholangitis due to a stone in the common bile duct should be suspected. The abdominal radiograph is normal; the majority of gallstones are radiolucent and do not show on plain films.

> **! DIFFERENTIAL DIAGNOSES**
>
> The major differential diagnoses of upper abdominal pain radiating to the back are:
> - Acute cholecystitis
> - Biliary colic
> - Perforated peptic ulcer
> - Acute pancreatitis
> - Acute hepatitis
> - Subphrenic abscess
> - Retrocaecal appendicitis
> - Right pyelonephritis
> - Perforated carcinoma or diverticulum of the hepatic flexure of the colon
> - Myocardial infarction or right lower lobe pneumonia may also mimic cholecystitis.

This patient should be admitted under the surgical team. Serum amylase should be measured to rule out pancreatitis. Blood cultures should be taken to guide antibiotic decisions. Chest radiograph should be performed to exclude pneumonia and erect abdominal radiograph to rule out air under the diaphragm, which occurs with a perforated peptic ulcer. An abdominal ultrasound will show gallstones and inflammation of the gallbladder wall. The patient should be kept nil by mouth, given intravenous fluids, analgesia and commenced on intravenous antibiotics. The patient should be examined regularly for signs of generalised peritonitis or cholangitis. If the symptoms subside, the patient is normally discharged to be readmitted in a few weeks once the inflammation has settled down to have a cholecystectomy. An immediate cholecystectomy may be considered in low-risk patients.

 KEY POINTS

- Acute cholecystitis typically causes right-upper-quadrant pain and a positive Murphy's sign.
- Potential complications include septicaemia and peritonitis.

CASE 97: WEIGHT LOSS

History

A 66-year-old retired nurse consults her general practitioner (GP) with a 4-month history of tiredness, slight breathlessness on exertion and loss of weight from 71 kg to 65 kg. Her appetite is unchanged and normal; she has no nausea or vomiting, but over the last 2 months, she has noticed a change in her bowel habit. She reports episodes of constipation alternating with her usual and normal pattern. She has not seen any blood in her faeces and has had no abdominal pain. She has had no postmenopausal bleeding. There is no relevant past or family history, and she is on no medication.

She has a 48 pack-year history and drinks 20–28 units of alcohol a week.

Examination

She has slight pallor but otherwise looks well. No lymphadenopathy is detected and her breasts, thyroid, heart, chest and abdomen, including rectal examination, are all normal. The blood pressure is 148/90 mmHg.

🔍 INVESTIGATIONS

		Normal
Haemoglobin	10.1 g/dL	11.7–15.7 g/dL
Mean corpuscular volume (MCV)	76 fL	80–99 fL
White cell count	4.9×10^9/L	$3.5–11.0 \times 10^9$/L
Platelets	277×10^9/L	$150–440 \times 10^9$/L
Sodium	142 mmol/L	135–145 mmol/L
Potassium	4.4 mmol/L	3.5–5.0 mmol/L
Urea	5.2 mmol/L	2.5–6.7 mmol/L
Creatinine	106 µmol/L	70–120 µmol/L

Urinalysis: no protein, no blood

Blood film shows a microcytic hypochromic picture.

❓ QUESTIONS

- What is the likeliest diagnosis?
- How would you investigate the patient?
- How can we screen for this condition?

ANSWER 97

The investigations show a microcytic, hypochromic anaemia. In a premenopausal woman, the most likely cause would be excessive menstrual blood loss. In men or postmenopausal women, the most likely cause would be loss from the gastrointestinal tract. This woman has an altered bowel habit, which suggests a problem with the lower gastrointestinal tract. Taking this into account, the most likely differential would be a carcinoma of the colon, which would also explain her weight loss. A barium enema revealed a neoplasm in the sigmoid colon, confirmed by colonoscopy and biopsy. Chest radiograph and abdominal ultrasound showed no pulmonary metastases and no intra-abdominal lymphadenopathy or hepatic metastases, respectively.

She proceeded to a sigmoid colectomy and end-to-end anastomosis and was regularly followed-up for any evidence of recurrence. Histology showed a stage I tumour.

Carcinoma of the colon is increasing in frequency. If it presents at an early stage, the prognosis is good. Rectal bleeding, alteration in bowel habit for longer than 1 month at any age or iron-deficient anaemia in men or postmenopausal women are indications for investigation of the gastrointestinal tract. In younger people, there may be a hereditary element to carcinoma of the colon.

Smoking is a risk factor for carcinoma of the colon.

Bowel cancer screening is offered to everyone aged 60 to 74 years in the UK and is expanding to ages 50 to 59 over the coming years. This home test kit, called a faecal immunochemical test (FIT), can detect occult blood in the faeces that may be an early sign of a carcinoma.

 KEY POINTS

- Carcinoma of the colon can present with few or no symptoms or signs in the gastrointestinal tract.
- Unexplained iron deficiency anaemia warrants investigation of the upper and lower gastrointestinal tract.

CASE 98: ABDOMINAL PAIN

History

A 31-year-old woman has a 6-year history of abdominal pain and bloating. She has had an irregular bowel habit with periods of increased bowel actions up to four times a day and periods of constipation. Opening her bowels tends to relieve the pain, which has been present in her lower abdomen. She had similar problems around the age of 17, which led to time off school. She thinks that her pains are made worse after eating citrus fruits and after some vegetables and wheat. She has tried to exclude these from her diet with some temporary relief, but overall there has been no change in the symptoms over the 6 years. One year ago, she was seen in a gastro-enterology clinic and had a sigmoidoscopy, which was normal. She found the procedure very uncomfortable and developed similar symptoms of abdominal pain during the procedure. She is anxious about the continuing pain but is not keen to have a further endoscopy.

She has a history of occasional episodes of headache, which have been diagnosed as migraine, and has irregular periods with troublesome period pains but no other relevant medical history. She is a non-smoker who does not drink alcohol. Her paternal grandmother died at age 64 years of carcinoma of the colon. Her parents are alive and well. She works as a secretary.

Examination

Examination of the cardiovascular and respiratory systems is normal. She has a palpable, rather tender colon in the left iliac fossa.

INVESTIGATIONS		
		Normal
Haemoglobin	11.9 g/dL	11.7–15.7 g/dL
Mean corpuscular volume (MCV)	84 fL	80–99 fL
White cell count	5.3×10^9/L	$3.5–11.0 \times 10^9$/L
Platelets	244×10^9/L	$150–440 \times 10^9$/L
Erythrocyte sedimentation rate (ESR)	8 mm/h	<10 mm/h
Sodium	138 mmol/L	135–145 mmol/L
Potassium	4.4 mmol/L	3.5–5.0 mmol/L
Urea	4.2 mmol/L	2.5–6.7 mmol/L
Creatinine	89 µmol/L	70–120 µmol/L
Glucose	4.6 mmol/L	4.0–6.0 mmol/L

? QUESTIONS

- What is the most likely diagnosis?
- What investigations should be performed?
- What treatment options are there for this patient?

ANSWER 98

The pattern of the pain, the absence of physical signs, normal investigations and reproduction of the pain during sigmoidoscopy all make it likely that this is irritable bowel syndrome (IBS). This is a very common condition accounting for a large number of referrals to gastroenterology clinics. IBS is often episodic, with variable periods of relapse and remission. Periods of frequent defaecation alternate with periods of relative constipation. Relapses are often associated with periods of stress. In IBS it is common to have a history of other conditions, such as migraine and menstrual irregularity. Under the age of 40 years with a history of 6 years of similar problems, it would be reasonable to accept the diagnosis and reassure the patient. However, the family history of carcinoma of the colon raises the possibility of a condition such as familial polyposis coli. The family history and the patient's feelings about this should be explored further. Anxiety about the family history might contribute to the patient's own symptoms or her presentation at this time. If there are living family members with polyposis coli, DNA probing may be used to identify family members at high risk. If any doubt remains, it would be sensible to proceed to a barium enema or a colonoscopy to rule out any significant problems.

The diagnosis of IBS relies on the exclusion of other significant conditions, such as inflammatory bowel disease, diverticular disease or large-bowel malignancy. In patients under the age of 40 years, it is usually reasonable to do this based on the history, examination and a normal full blood count and ESR. In older patients, a sigmoidoscopy and barium enema or colonoscopy should be performed. First-line management should be according to the predominant symptoms. Pain may be helped by antispasmodic drugs, constipation may require laxatives and diarrhoea can be helped with loperamide. Second-line pharmacological treatment includes tricyclic antidepressants. Psychological interventions such as cognitive behavioural therapy may also be beneficial.

 KEY POINTS

- Irritable bowel syndrome is a common disorder and difficult to treat.
- Explanation of the condition to the patient is an important part of the management.
- Sigmoidoscopy with air insufflation often reproduces the symptoms of IBS.

CASE 99: ABDOMINAL PAIN

History

A 74-year-old woman has a 10-year history of intermittent lower abdominal pain. The pain has been colicky in nature and is associated with a feeling of distension in the left iliac fossa. It is generally relieved by passing flatus or faeces. She tends to be constipated and passes small pieces of faeces. Four years previously, she passed some blood with her stools and had a barium enema performed. The radiograph of this is shown in Figure 99.1. Over the past week, her pain has worsened and now she has continuous pain in the left iliac fossa and feels generally unwell. Her appetite has been poor over this same time. She has not had her bowels open over the last 2 days. In her previous medical history, she had a hysterectomy for fibroids 20 years ago. There is a family history of ischaemic heart disease and diabetes mellitus. She lives alone and does her own cooking and shopping.

Examination

She has a temperature of 38.5°C and her abdomen is tender with a vague impression of a mass in the left iliac fossa. There is no guarding or rebound tenderness and the bowel sounds are normal. Her pulse is 84/min, and blood pressure is 154/88 mmHg. No abnormalities are found in the respiratory system.

🔍 INVESTIGATIONS

		Normal
Haemoglobin	11.8 g/dL	11.7–15.7 g/dL
Mean corpuscular volume (MCV)	85 fL	80–99 fL
White cell count	15.6×10^9/L	$3.5–11.0 \times 10^9$/L
Platelets	235×10^9/L	$150–440 \times 10^9$/L
C-reactive protein (CRP)	56 mg/L	<5 mg/L

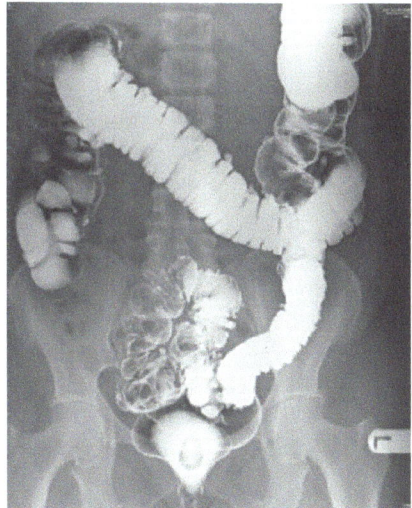

❓ QUESTIONS

- What is the likely diagnosis?
- What should be the initial management?
- What management should be considered long term?

Figure 99.1 Barium enema.

DOI: 10.1201/9781003350934-109

ANSWER 99

This woman has diverticulitis. Colonic diverticula are small outpouchings that are most commonly found in the left colon. They are very common in the elderly Western population, likely associated with a deficiency in dietary fibre. Symptomatic diverticular disease has many of the features of irritable bowel syndrome. Inflammation in a diverticulum is termed diverticulitis. In severe cases, perforation, paracolic abscess formation or septicaemia may develop. Other potential complications include bowel obstruction, formation of a fistula into the rectum or vagina, and haemorrhage.

The barium enema from four years ago shows evidence of diverticular disease with outpouchings of the mucosa in the sigmoid colon. This would be consistent with the long-standing history of abdominal pain and constipation. The recent problems of increased pain, tenderness, fever, raised white cell count and CRP and a mass in the left iliac fossa would be compatible with an acute exacerbation of her diverticular disease. In this case, there is no evidence of peritonitis, which would signal a possible perforation of one of the diverticula.

The differential diagnosis, with the suggestion of a mass and change in bowel habit, would be carcinoma of the colon or Crohn's disease. Examination to rule out perforation with leak of bowel contents into the peritoneum (no peritonitis) and obstruction (normal bowel sounds, no general distension) is necessary. A computed tomography (CT) scan of the abdomen will delineate the mass and suggest whether there is evidence of local abscess or fistula formation.

Treatment should include broad-spectrum antibiotics (ciprofloxacin and metronidazole), intravenous fluids and rest. Further investigations are indicated, including urea and electrolytes, creatinine, glucose values, liver function tests and blood cultures. A colonoscopy should be performed at a later date to exclude the possibility of a colonic neoplasm.

Repeated severe episodes, bleeding or obstruction may require surgical intervention. Patients are advised to eat a high-fibre diet once the acute episode has subsided.

 KEY POINTS

- Diverticular disease is a common finding in the elderly Western population and may be asymptomatic or cause irritable bowel syndrome-type symptoms.
- Diverticular disease is a common condition; its presence can distract the unwary doctor from pursuing a coincident condition.
- Diverticulitis needs to be treated with antibiotics to reduce the chance of complications occurring, such as perforation or fistula formation.

History

A 34-year-old woman presents to her general practitioner (GP) to discuss a rash that has developed over the past 2 weeks. There are multiple tender red swellings on her shins and forearms. The older swellings are darker in colour and seem to be healing from the centre. She feels generally unwell and tired and has pain in her wrists and ankles. Over the past 2 years she has had recurrent aphthous ulcers in her mouth. She has had no genital ulceration, but she has been troubled by intermittent abdominal pain and diarrhoea. She works as a waitress and is unmarried. She smokes about 15 cigarettes per day and drinks alcohol only occasionally. She has no other previous medical illnesses, and there is no relevant family history that she can recall.

Examination

She is thin but looks well. There are no aphthous ulcers to see at the time of the examination. Her joints are not inflamed, and the range of movement is not restricted or painful. Examining the skin, there are multiple tender lesions on the shins and forearms. The lesions are raised and vary from 1 cm to 3 cm in diameter. The fresher lesions are red, and the older ones look like bruises. Physical examination is otherwise normal.

INVESTIGATIONS

		Normal
Haemoglobin	13.5 g/dL	11.7–15.7 g/dL
White cell count	15.4 × 10⁹/L	3.5–11.0 × 10⁹/L
Platelets	198 × 10⁹/L	150–440 × 10⁹/L
Erythrocyte sedimentation rate (ESR)	98 mm/h	<10 mm/h
Sodium	138 mmol/L	135–145 mmol/L
Potassium	4.3 mmol/L	3.5–5.0 mmol/L
Urea	5.4 mmol/L	2.5–6.7 mmol/L
Creatinine	86 µmol/L	70–120 µmol/L
Glucose	5.8 mmol/L	4.0–6.0 mmol/L

Chest radiograph: normal

Urinalysis: normal

QUESTIONS

- What is the diagnosis?
- What are the major causes of this condition?
- How would you manage this patient?

DOI: 10.1201/9781003350934-110

ANSWER 100

This patient has erythema nodosum, in this case, secondary to previously undiagnosed Crohn's disease. Erythema nodosum is due to inflammation of the small blood vessels in the deep dermis. Characteristically, it affects the shins, but it may also affect the thighs and forearms. The number and size of the lesions vary. Lesions tend to heal from the centre and spread peripherally. The rash is often preceded by systemic symptoms—fever, malaise and arthralgia. It usually resolves over 3–4 weeks, but persistence or recurrence suggests an underlying disease.

 DISEASES LINKED TO ERYTHEMA NODOSUM

Streptococcal infection	Lymphoma/leukaemia
Tuberculosis	Sarcoidosis
Leprosy	Pregnancy/oral contraceptive
Glandular fever	Reaction to sulphonamides
Histoplasmosis	Ulcerative colitis
Coccidioidomycosis	Crohn's disease

The history of mouth ulcers, abdominal pain and diarrhoea strongly suggests that this woman has Crohn's disease. She should therefore be referred to a gastroenterologist for investigations, which should include a small-bowel enema and colonoscopy with biopsies. Treatment of her underlying disease with steroids should cause the erythema nodosum to resolve. With no serious underlying condition, erythema nodosum usually settles with non-steroidal anti-inflammatory drugs.

🔑 **KEY POINTS**

- Patients presenting with erythema nodosum should be investigated for an underlying disease.
- Erythema nodosum is most often seen on the shins but can affect the extensor surface of the forearms or thighs.

INDEX

Note: *Italic* page numbers refer to *figures*.

D

E

F

G

H

Q

R

S

X

Z